ESTHER YODER

nourish

nour-ish [nur-ish] v.

- To sustain with food or nutriment; supply with what is necessary for life, health, and growth.
- To cherish, stimulate, or nurture
- To strengthen, support

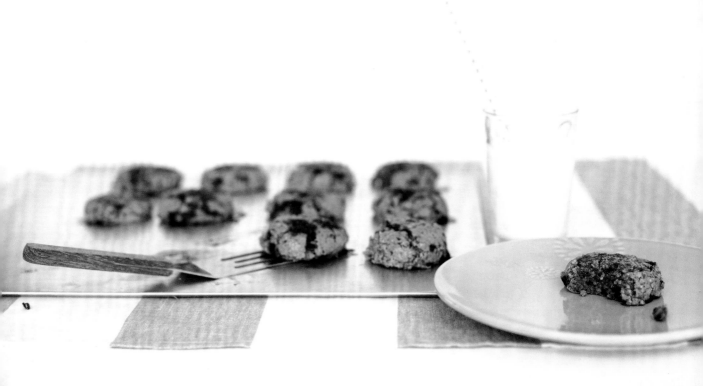

nourish✗cook

Copyright © 2014 by Nourish Cook

THIS BOOK IS DEDICATED TO OUR SWEET DAUGHTER, ANDRIA, AND TO INDIVIDUALS EVERYWHERE WITH EPILEPSY.

LOW GLYCEMIC INDEX DIET:

A carbohydrate-controlled diet, utilizing low glycemic carbohydrates, with an emphasis on fats and adequate protein intake.

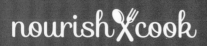

contents

BEVERAGES, HORS D'OEUVRES & SNACKS......................17–50

BREAKFAST & BREADS..51–65

SOUPS & SALADS...66–88

PANINIS, QUESADILLAS & WRAPS.............................89–99

MAIN DISHES & SIDES..100–132

BAKE SHOP DESSERTS..133–165

CONFECTIONERY...166–174

THE HOME PANTRY: PRESERVES & MIXES................175–186

INDEX..188–189

SOURCES...189

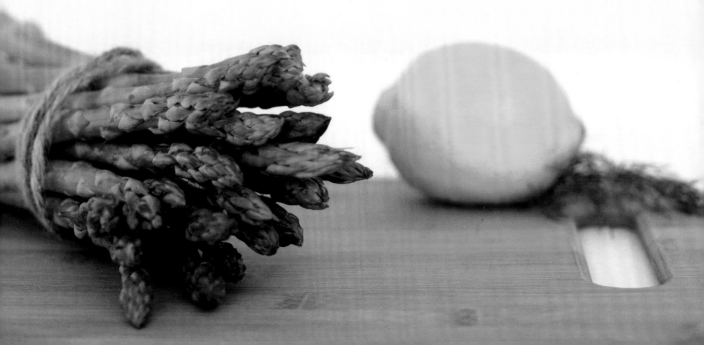

FOREWORD

A MESSAGE FROM OUR DOCTOR

Dietary therapy has long been used in a wide variety of medical ailments. There has been interest in the last several years in using low glycemic index diets to reduce obesity and obesity related health risk factors. Numerous recent studies have shown a clear improvement in obesity and cholesterol in those who follow a low glycemic index diet. This particular diet has also been investigated more recently as an option to improve the lives of patients with epilepsy. Our authors, whose journey with epilepsy began with their daughter only a few short years ago, were compelled to explore this diet as a natural regimen to try to improve her life, and they succeeded!

Of neurological disorders, epilepsy continues to be a difficult and unpredictable entity for adults, children, their families, and the medical professionals who help care for these individuals. The beneficial effect of specific diets in patients with epilepsy has been documented for centuries. A renewed interest in dietary therapy for epilepsy is evident in medical literature as early as the 1920's. In the last decade, the Low Glycemic Index Diet has had a significant surge of interest in its use for patients who do not achieve control of their seizures adequately with medications, surgery, or the combination of the two.

This collection fills a need for those individuals and families who wish to explore the Low Glycemic Index Diet and provides over one hundred easy-to-follow recipes for both convenience and variety. My hope is that this compilation, so graciously and diligently prepared by the Yoder family, will help those looking for a natural alternative to improve their health and quality of life!

Esther, James, and Andria have all given of themselves to see this book come to fruition. We admire their perseverance, patience, and continued belief that food can be more than just nutrition.

Practicing Pediatric Epilepsy Specialist

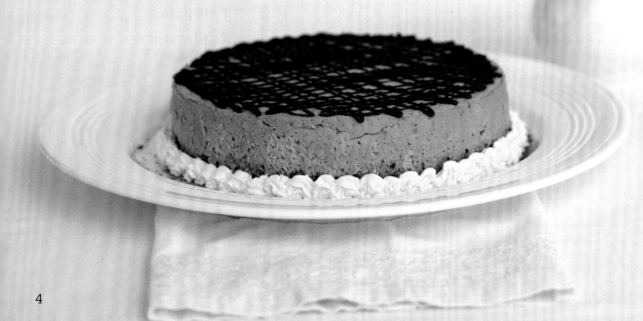

4

INTRODUCTION

Welcome to the world of low glycemic index cooking! A world where creativity has boundless opportunity, and where the sky is the limit on the imaginative use of food and ingredients. A world where necessity becomes the mother of success. I would like to share our story as an introduction to this cookbook.

Three years ago, our daughter Andria, then 4, was diagnosed with absence seizures. Thus began our long journey with anti-seizure medication.

The first drug we tried seemed to be a disaster from day one, as we were seeing no let up in seizures, and it made Andria feel awful.

The second choice was better, but the side effects were still quite pronounced. Andria became very lethargic and irritable, as well as uncommunicative and unresponsive. Physically, her balance was poor, along with regression and shakiness in fine motor skills. I remember seeing her at mealtime struggling to eat neatly, and finding difficult even the simple act of drinking from a glass without spilling water. As any parent will understand, seeing medication completely change one's child into someone you hardly recognize is very, very difficult. So, although we felt the seizures were controlled, it seemed to be a poor exchange for what the medicine was doing to her body.

The third medicine seemed a bit better, but we were continually increasing the dosage. Seizures were absent for up to two months after a medicine increase, then suddenly we would see them again every day. More medicine. And more medicine. The levels were disturbingly high as our sweet little girl was changed into a person we hardly knew.

AN ALTERNATIVE SOLUTION

In the world of pediatric neurology, we were working with Dr. Stephen Fulton and a clinical dietitian, Rebecca Jennings, at the Le Bonheur Children's Hospital in Memphis. We came to respect Dr. Fulton's advice and opinion deeply through this time, as we sensed a genuine and personal interest in seeing our daughter become seizure free. Because of Andria's unsatisfactory response to medicine in general, he suggested trying the Low Glycemic Index Diet as an alternative seizure control method. Initially, we were excited about a diet; however, as we researched and learned the implications this would have on our lifestyle and eating, we became very cautious. As we discussed it at length, our apprehension deepened. Could we do this? After weighing our remaining options, which at this point were very limited, we decided to take the plunge.

BEGINNING THE DIET

With that decision, our world of "normal" living and eating did a complete metamorphosis. The plain, raw truth was that I was completely unprepared for the upheaval in Andria's eating habits. As Andria's parents, my husband and I were dedicated to the best treatment available for our daughter, although it meant sacrifice on our part. Being united in the decision to go ahead with the diet was one of our strongest assets. The diet itself was a completely new world as I discovered that even foods I considered to be "healthy" were off limits. Armed with a list of acceptable foods and sample menus, I was skeptical as to which of those foods Andria would actually eat. That list was frighteningly short.

To my advantage, I have been cooking since I could follow a recipe, so the kitchen was familiar territory. To our disadvantage, we have a strong culture of sharing food and mealtime with family and friends, and lots of home-style cooking. So, although junk food and fast food weren't a huge part of our lifestyle, neither was our cooking altogether healthy. My pantry was well-stocked with white sugar, white flour, and all the yummy, not-good-for-you ingredients that can be turned into luscious, carbohydrate-laden comfort foods. I was quite inexperienced in the art of food label reading and would hardly have known a carbohydrate if I had met one on the street. So, yes, the journey was long and the learning curve was gigantic!

Time was another issue with which I battled. We had three young children at the time, and my days were already full to overflowing with the busyness of living. Amazingly, after taking the initial leap, time seemed to make itself, as I made it a priority to have healthy food available each day.

I'm not going to pretend this diet was easy! At the beginning, it was extremely stressful. When we made the decision to do it as a three month trial, we resolved we were going to do it right, or not at all. The first week was nothing less than a mother's nightmare, as I scrambled for ideas and fumbled my way through new foods. Now I was the mommy standing in the aisle at the supermarket intently reading food labels. I was the one lying awake at night unable to stop the relentless march of an over-worked brain.

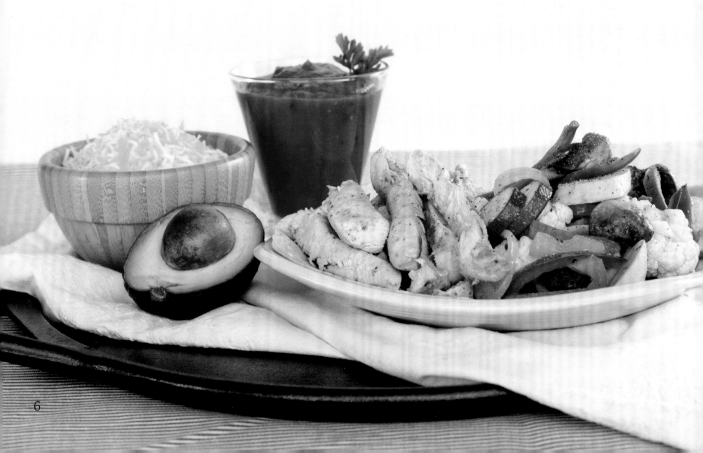

ASSISTANCE AND PROGRESSION

There were several factors during this time that carried us through, the largest being our faith. We felt that through Dr. Fulton, God had brought this plan of possible healing to us, and so we trusted and prayed our way through the difficulties. My husband's unwavering support helped carry me through the times I felt completely burned out. Being further removed from the situation helped him step in with new tactics and fresh food ideas. Rebecca Jennings, our dietitian, was very patient and tireless with our long lists of questions.

The really good news is that this became much, much easier. The more I became familiar with the diet, the more things came together in my mind, and it all started to make sense. In my constant quest, I was discovering new foods every day, and ideas began to flow as I worked among my pots and pans. I saw this was going to be a great place to get creative with foods, seasonings, and cooking methods.

At our three month follow-up doctor visit, we had decreased medicine once and were seeing no seizures. We agreed to stay on the Low Glycemic Index Diet for the long haul if Andria continued doing well. We had gone from a trial period to a long-term lifestyle change. We were confident this was something we wanted to pursue for the health of our daughter.

SUCCESS

In the months following, the results of the diet were amazing. As we successfully began to decrease Andria's Lamictal dosage, I became focused on seeing the food on her plate at mealtime as her medicine. My mentality of food and the purpose of eating completely changed. While I previously saw meals as social and pleasurable events, I now also viewed them as important sources of nourishment. As refined and processed foods were eliminated, and fresh, whole foods were used instead, we saw the positive impact on Andria's body.

We went with a schedule of reducing meds every six weeks, and saw incredible changes. First, there was absolutely no more seizure activity. Ever. That is how well the diet worked as seizure control. That we had gone from a steadily increasing medicine dosage to a steady decrease felt nothing short of miraculous. The negative side effects were rapidly disappearing, and our active, happy child was returning. Andria was in first grade in school and coming home consistently with straight A's.

In August of 2013, after one year of being on the diet, Andria was seizure and medicine free. We felt blessed to have our prayers answered in this way, and very grateful to Dr. Fulton for introducing us to this method of treatment. In my mind's eye, I can clearly recall a memory of Andria after ten months of being on the diet. I was walking in the lane after an evening stroll, and she came to meet me. Imagine a little girl, flying along on her bike, with rosy cheeks and brown eyes sparkling with laughter. It was a picture of radiance and health. In that moment, I remembered the lethargic, sad, pale child she used to be, and realized the true effects of the Low Glycemic Index Diet!

THE CHALLENGES AND OUR SECRETS TO SUCCESS

Along the journey, we have uncovered a wealth of information which has made life manageable and doable for our family. I feel light-years ahead of where I was when I began this method of cooking. The frantic despair and moments of panic have been replaced with the confidence of a solid course of action. Compiling this cookbook has become a work of the heart as I share the things that paved the way for us to a new kind of normal. Although we had phenomenal success with diet therapy in treating epilepsy, it is not a solution for everyone. However, our goal for this book is that more children like Andria can become seizure free, as well as medicine free.

Our extended families and friends have been an awesome support group, especially in sharing recipes and ideas from their kitchens that could be incorporated into Andria's everyday menus. Small acts of thoughtfulness would bring sunshine into a difficult day. Friends of ours cured ham and bacon with no nitrates or carbohydrates especially for Andria. Another friend gifted us with farm fresh poultry.

Because we used the Low Glycemic Index Diet as a seizure control treatment for our young daughter, I have geared my recipes toward child friendly meals. As you acclimate and become more informed, allow yourself to expand the variety of dishes—within the limits of the diet, of course.

PREPARATION FOR THE DIET

My most important recommendation in starting the diet is to plan ahead. I see that if I had done this before we actually plunged into the diet, it would have eliminated much of the stress. Beginning with a list of foods you are confident your child will eat, make a list of menus for the first two weeks. Now start cooking! Invest in small one cup plastic or glass containers that can be stored in the freezer and marked with the contents and the carb amounts. When cooking one dish, make enough for six servings. Keep one in the refrigerator, and freeze the rest. This saves an incredible amount of time! Just the knowledge of having backup meals in the freezer is a great relief for the busier days when there is no time to cook. Expect to have lots of trial and error in the beginning—both in your food preparation and as you learn what foods your child will enjoy or reject.

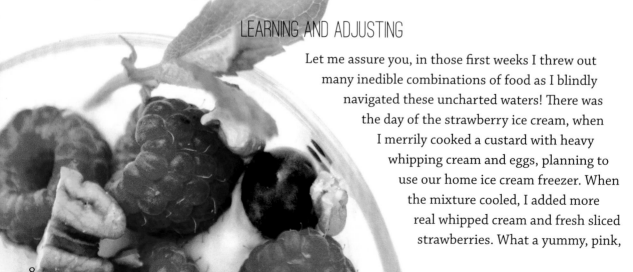

LEARNING AND ADJUSTING

Let me assure you, in those first weeks I threw out many inedible combinations of food as I blindly navigated these uncharted waters! There was the day of the strawberry ice cream, when I merrily cooked a custard with heavy whipping cream and eggs, planning to use our home ice cream freezer. When the mixture cooled, I added more real whipped cream and fresh sliced strawberries. What a yummy, pink, cloud-like concoction I was turning out! Just before freezing, I tasted it and ugh! I had used stevia as a sweetener and had used roughly ten times the amount I should have. I took the entire bowl out the back door and dumped it into the dog's dish. Our dog ate well those first few weeks!

When a food did turn out well, but Andria turned up her nose, I put it away and reintroduced it later. As she adjusted to new tastes and ways of eating, many of those things eventually became her favorites. For example, one of my big concerns before starting the diet was that Andria was not a meat lover. She would push that portion of her meal all over her plate before taking tiny nibbles. Guess what? Today Andria loves meat! She will sit at the table with only meat on her plate and inhale it. Don't rush the adjustment process—adapting takes time!

SERVING SIZES AND SWEETENERS

Portion control and serving sizes are another part of the learning curve. Invest in two sets of stackable measuring cups if you don't already have them. In addition to the extra cooking, there will be measuring for serving size. One advantage to a child on the diet, is that the portions can naturally be smaller, thus allowing for some special foods in small amounts. For instance, we bought low carb ice cream and used it only on weekends or when we had guests at our house. I served it in half serving size portions, making this a great little treat for her. Because Andria was a born snacker, I found it paid to keep her mealtime carbs absolutely as low as possible, giving us more room to work in snacks.

Sweeteners are another enormous issue. I use liquid sucralose in beverages and in whipped cream, where the flavor is the most prominent. Stevia works better in cooking and baking, and I find liquid stevia to be a bit less concentrated or bitter than the powdered stevia, although I use both. Know that these sugar substitutes never give the food that truly "sweet" taste that comes when using sugar. Adding too much sucralose or stevia will produce a bitter or sour aftertaste.

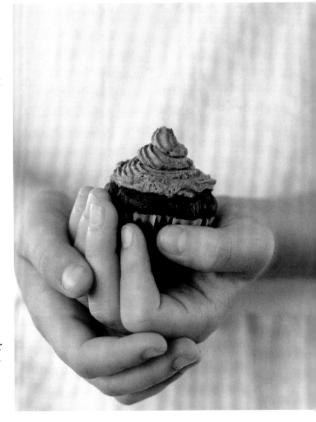

THE GOOD STUFF

The freedom to liberally use butter and heavy whipping cream is a great bonus in enhancing otherwise bland foods with flavor and richness. Make the most of this advantage. Adding cheese was another sure way to top off entrées successfully.

Another big discovery in this department was using cocoa, spices (e.g. cinnamon or nutmeg), and other seasonings instead of sweeteners. Be prepared to season or flavor foods rather than sweetening them. With a bit of experimenting you may be pleasantly surprised! Taste as you mix a recipe, adding or subtracting as desired.

Think of the recipes as a loose guide as you go along, making changes with the seasoning amounts to fit your likes and dislikes.

SUPPLEMENTS

Getting Andria to take her daily vitamins was another hurdle that caused lots of trouble in the beginning. She was taking adult-sized vitamins as a supplement to the diet, so I was crushing and mixing the powder with food. As you can imagine, that did not produce a desirable taste in any circumstance. There are several newer products available now in a powder version for ease of administration. These can be mixed into liquids or sugar free Jell-O®.

Another issue that produced much trouble was constipation. We turned to Miralax® for help, which in turn produced more pain. I found a natural product from Integrative Therapeutics®; a liquid calcium magnesium 1:1 ratio. We worked out an appropriate dosage with our dietitian, and it radically helped with the constipation. Counting the extra carbohydrate it contained turned out to be easier than dealing with constant discomfort.

MOTIVATION

As I mentioned earlier, I was at an advantage because I had been cooking almost all my life. If this is a new realm for you, it's not too late to learn! Start at the beginning with simple things and work your way up. Having said that, don't hesitate to ask for assistance if you are in over your head. We had an allergy-friendly baker who came to the farmer's market every week. She was a great source of knowledge and especially focused on helping children with special diets. Finding someone like this to help can be a lifeline to sanity.

One of the most rewarding parts of doing your own cooking is the connection that develops with the ingredients you use. This allows you to know what is in the food you eat. The simple act of preparing your own food can change your life, creating a sense of control over what you are ingesting. This power and knowledge will enable you to not only feed yourself and your family, but to truly nourish well.

Factors Influencing Glycemic Index	
Cooking Time	*Longer cooking times tend to raise the glycemic index of foods because carbohydrates are broken down and are more easily absorbed by the body.*
Fiber	*Fiber is a type of carbohydrate that slows down digestion and is not readily absorbed thereby lowering the glycemic index of a meal.*
Acidity	*Adding acidic foods, such as lemon juice or vinegar, will lower glycemic index.*
Food Combinations	*Protein and fats, when combined with carbohydrates, will lower the glycemic impact of a meal.*

A NOTE FROM OUR DIETITIAN

This is a carbohydrate-controlled, low glycemic cookbook compiled by Esther Yoder for her daughter Andria. Andria suffers from seizures and her doctor recommended the Low Glycemic Index Diet as another tool in her treatment. Always consult your doctor before making any changes to a medical treatment plan, including the addition of nutrition therapy.

BACKGROUND OF DIET THERAPY FOR SEIZURES

The idea of diet therapy to treat illness and for long term health is not new. Think of the age-old Hippocrates saying "Let food be thy medicine and medicine be thy food." But you may be surprised to know that diet can be one of the most effective treatments for difficult to control seizures in children. Ketogenic diets have been used since the 1920's to effectively treat many different types of seizures. The ketogenic diet is an extremely high fat, low carbohydrate diet meant to switch the body's main fuel source from carbohydrates to dietary fats. When the body breaks down fat for energy, you get ketones. It is estimated that 2 out of 3 children with seizures who attempt the ketogenic diet see a 50% or greater reduction in their seizures, with a fortunate few becoming seizure free. Despite the diet's successful use for nearly a century, we still do not completely understand how the diet works in regards to seizure control. In other words, we don't know why it works. It just works.

But the ketogenic diet is no picnic. It is labor-intensive and not without side effects. All meals must be carefully calculated to a prescribed ketogenic ratio, and all foods weighed on a gram scale. The ketogenic diet can also be unappetizing and socially isolating, making long-term compliance difficult. Potential side effects include low blood sugar, constipation, acidosis, high triglycerides/cholesterol, altered growth and kidney stones. Other simplified versions of the ketogenic diet have emerged to combat some of these issues. One such version is the Low Glycemic Index Diet for seizures developed by Dr. Elizabeth Thiele and dietitian Heidi Pfeifer from Massachusetts General Hospital in Boston. Their results were first published in 2005.

ABOUT THE LOW GLYCEMIC INDEX DIET FOR SEIZURES *(see chart on opposite page)*

The goal of the Low Glycemic Index Diet is to lower and stabilize the blood sugar throughout the day. This, in theory, limits stimulation in the brain via decreased glucose metabolism and/or hormonal changes, which may be linked with seizure control in affected children or adults. The functional mechanism has not been fully explained.

The Low Glycemic Index Diet is **not** intended to induce ketosis. A Low Glycemic Index Diet for seizures is designed to be low in carbohydrates and higher in protein and fats. In addition to the amount of carbohydrates, the type of carbohydrate also needs to be considered. The carbohydrates used should have a low glycemic index score and are measured by using simple kitchen tools like measuring cups and spoons. Glycemic index is a measure of how much a carbohydrate containing food raises blood sugar. Foods are scored from 1–100, with 100 being a reference food such as sugar (i.e. glucose.) A low glycemic index food will have a score less than 50. There are many factors which will influence a food's glycemic

index. These include cooking time, fiber, acidity and food combinations. It can be a challenge to locate the glycemic index
of certain carbohydrate containing foods and information can
vary by source. Cue the Yoder family.

MEETING THE YODERS

I first met Andria Yoder in the summer of 2012. She is
a miniature version of her charming mother, Esther. Diet
therapy was discussed as a possible treatment for Andria in
the past and this was met with some apprehension, verging
on shock and horror. You can read more from Esther's point of
view in her introduction.

This is a natural reaction when you ask anyone to change
what and how they eat, especially with our food focused culture. There was much to consider. Would Andria feel "different" from everyone else? Is the diet healthy? What about the
possible side effects? Would she gain weight? Would she lose
weight? What about follow-up labs and doctor's visits? Not
easy for a family who lives several hours away. And, not to
be left out, would Andria ever be able to enjoy sweets again?
These are all important questions to discuss with your doctor and dietitian when considering any special
diet. But, when faced with Andria's negative experience with multiple medicines, the Yoders decided it
was time to give the Low Glycemic Index Diet a try.

The Yoders and I sat down in our first meeting and talked about the diet plan, possible side effects and
expected follow-up. They were provided food lists, a sample menu, a list of required nutritional supplements and dietitian contact information. At the end of that first meeting, we shook hands, "Have a nice
day," "Please call or email with any questions." It was a routine visit.

The next day, Esther had a few questions. OK, more than a few. And I'm glad she did. Esther really
made us think about the diet and what a family needs in order to be successful with a low glycemic diet
in the "real world." Many emails were exchanged wherein we discussed different foods, discerning what
would be allowed and what would need to be avoided. Maybe a food had a high glycemic index, or this
one was low glycemic index but too high in carbohydrates and would need to be avoided. Maybe a food
item did not have a glycemic index score, but it was overall low carbohydrate and high fiber and was
deemed acceptable. We were also struggling to find resources that were relevant for the Low Glycemic
Index Diet for seizures, which is not only low glycemic, but also low carbohydrate.

Once the Yoder family saw the diet was helping to control Andria's seizures, they wanted to help other
families who were embarking on a similar journey. Esther saw the need for a child friendly, low glycemic,
low carbohydrate resource, which would be applicable for children (and adults) and that is just what she

Guide to the
NUTRITIONAL FACTS

Serving Size The amount of a
single serving.
Calories The amount of energy
from a single serving.
Total Fat Fats generally lower the
glycemic impact of a meal due to
slower stomach emptying.
Total Carbohydrate Includes
starches, sugar and fiber. Carbohydrates will raise blood sugar and are
limited to 40-60 grams per day on
the Low Glycemic Diet for seizures.
Dietary Fiber Aim for foods high
in fiber.
Sugar Aim for foods low in sugar.
Protein Proteins generally lower
the glycemic impact of a meal due to
slower stomach emptying.

has created. This book can be the greatest tool in the kitchen when starting out on the Low Glycemic Index Diet. No culinary training needed, just an open mind. Bon appétit!

Rebecca Jennings, MS, RD
Clinical Pediatric Dietitian at Le Bonheur Children's Hospital
Memphis, Tennessee

Summary of the Low Glycemic Index Diet for Seizures
- Developed by Dr. Elizabeth Thiele and dietitian Heidi Pfeifer from Massachusetts General Hospital and first published in 2005.
- Low in carbohydrates, with a glycemic index less than 50.
- The diet should be discussed with your doctor to determine if it is appropriate.
- Meet with a dietitian to determine appropriate calorie, carbohydrate and protein goals as well as vitamin and mineral supplements needed to ensure the diet is complete.
- Potential side effects are similar to those for the classic ketogenic diet, though less likely to occur. They include low blood sugar, constipation, acidosis, high triglycerides/cholesterol, altered growth and kidney stones.
- Low Glycemic Index Diet can be used in children and adults, but will not work for everyone.
- Low Glycemic Index Diets have been studied in other conditions such as weight loss, diabetes and heart disease. New areas of research for low carbohydrate diets include cancer, Alzheimer's, autism and traumatic brain injury.

Selected References And Resources
Pfeifer HH, Thiele EA. Low-Glycemic-Index Treatment: A Liberalized Ketogenic Diet for Treatment of Intractable Epilepsy. *Neurology* 2005; 65: 1810-1812.
Pfeifer HH, Lyczkowski DA, Thiele EA. Low Glycemic Index Treatment: Implementation and New Insights into Efficacy. *Epilepsia* 2008; 49 (suppl. 8): 42-45.
Ketogenic Diets; Treatments for Epilepsy and Other Disorders.
Eric H. Kossoff, MD, John M. Freeman, MD, Zahava Turner, RD, CSP, LDN, and James E. Rubenstein, MD. Fifth Edition. Demos Medical Publishing, 2011.
The CalorieKing Calorie, Fat and Carbohydrate Counter 2013. Family Health Publications, Costa Mesa, CA, 2011. www.calorieking.com, 2013.
The Charlie Foundation to Help Cure Pediatric Epilepsy. www.charliefoundation.org, 2012.
Sydney University GI Research Service. www.glycemicindex.com, 2012.
U.S. Department of Agriculture, Agricultural Research Service. 2012. USDA National Nutrient Database for Standard Reference, Release 25. Nutrient Data Laboratory Home. www.ars.usda.gov/ba/bhnrc/ndl, 2012.

NUTRITION INFORMATION *Nutrition information is included for each recipe for your reference. Nutritional data was obtained from The USDA National Nutrient Database for Standard Reference and when applicable, from the specific brands utilized by the author in her recipes. Please be certain to refer to the food labels of the specific foods available in your area to ensure an accurate carbohydrate count. If you have questions about whether a food item is appropriate, consult with a dietitian.*

THE BASIC PRODUCTS AND INGREDIENTS TO GET STARTED

In addition to the list below, only the basic kitchen/pantry items generally used in cooking and baking are needed. Different brands of ingredients may have various performances when used in cooking and baking. Your first experiment with a recipe may not be perfect, but it will not be your last. The "practice makes perfect" rule applies very well to time spent in the kitchen. In the back of this book, I have included a list of sources that I have personally found to be the best place to purchase specialty ingredients.

NATURAL ALMOND MEAL This is the best flour substitute with the absolute lowest carb numbers that I have found. I recommend buying in 5 or 10 pound amounts, then storing in the freezer. I found the natural almond meal from Nickel Mine Health Foods to be the best in performance and price effectiveness. (see Sources)

SPROUTED WHEAT FLOUR Although this flour has a low glycemic index, the carbs are much higher than the almond meal. It carries a strong advantage of containing gluten, so it will imitate white and whole wheat flours more closely. I learned to use mostly almond meal with a very small amount of sprouted wheat flour in baking. (see Sources)

LIQUID SUCRALOSE Although initially this will take a bit of adjusting to taste, it is the sweetener of choice in beverages and whipped cream. (see Sources)

STEVIA This is a natural herb harvested from a plant and is extremely concentrated. It is an excellent choice for the Low Glycemic Index Diet, as it has no calories or carbs, and does not affect the blood sugar in any way. Use only in minutely small amounts, and experiment until you find what's right for you. I use both the powder and the liquid, although the powder seems to be the most concentrated.

AGAVE NECTAR Also considered low glycemic, agave nectar can be misleading because of the carbs. I use it only in one teaspoon amounts in recipes where I need to mimic the chemical properties of sugar.

XANTHAN GUM When mixed with liquid, xanthan gum forms an elastic texture which mimics gluten, making it an excellent choice when using almond meal. I recommend using only Bob's Red Mill®. (see Sources)

PURE VANILLA EXTRACT I love the difference in taste and quality when using pure vanilla extract. I use clear imitation vanilla flavoring only in recipes where the dark coloring of the pure vanilla is undesirable.

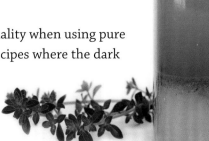

THE KITCHEN AND TOOLS

No fancy equipment is required for low glycemic cooking. The basic utensils found in any kitchen will do, but due to the higher volume of cooking, you may want to upgrade some items. For instance, I bought my third set of measuring spoons because I needed a 1/8 teaspoon measure. I would also recommend having two sets of measuring cups. There are definitely ways to streamline your time in the kitchen.

COOKWARE It pays to invest in high quality cookware. Although it's not imperative to purchase an entire set, my most-used pieces are as follows: a 6" nonstick skillet for sautéing, a 1 quart saucepan, and a 2 or 3 quart saucepan or Dutch oven. The Dutch oven will allow you to go from stove top to oven in one dish.

MIXER I use my KitchenAid® nearly every day. I also have a hand mixer that I use for small jobs.

IMMERSION BLENDER I love this handy tool! Every cook's nightmare of lumpy "anything" can be turned into something smooth and creamy. I especially use it with hot foods, placing the blender directly into the kettle.

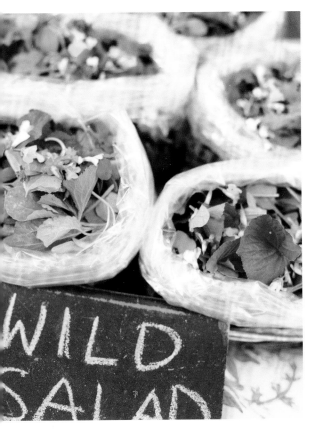

FOOD PROCESSOR OR BLENDER Although my kitchen is equipped with both of these appliances, I reach for my traditional style blender much more often. This is just a personal preference, because I have a glass pitcher attachment and can easily do hot or cold liquids in a flash, as well as crush ice for slushy drinks.

MINI FOOD CHOPPER Also indispensable for doing small jobs fast, I use the mini chopper for onions, bread crumbs, and much more.

SMALL KITCHEN SCALES This is not a must-have, but I found it very helpful when calculating carbs in foods difficult to measure in cups or tablespoons.

FREEZER With purchasing specialty food items and extra meal preparation, adequate freezer space is important. This also allows you to buy meat in bulk at lower prices.

LOW GLYCEMIC SHOPPING LIST

VEGETABLES

› Asparagus
› Bamboo Shoots
› Broccoli
› Brussels Sprouts
› Cabbage
› Carrots
› Cauliflower
› Celery
› Cucumbers
› Egg Plant
› Green Beans
› Jicama
› Kale
› Leeks
› Lettuce
› Mushrooms
› Onions
› Peppers
› Pickles
› Radish
› Salsa
› Sauerkraut
› Spinach
› Sprouts (*bean, alfalfa, broccoli*)
› Summer Squash
› Tomatoes
› Tomato Juice
› Zucchini

FRUITS

› Apples
› Apricots
› Avocados
› Blueberries
› Coconut
› Grapefruit
› Lemons
› Oranges
› Peaches
› Pears
› Raspberries
› Strawberries
› Blackberries

GRAINS AND STARCHES

› Beans
› Lentils
› Low-Carb Whole Grain Flatbread With Flax
› Low-Carb Whole Grain Tortilla
› Pearled Barley
› Sprouted Whole Grain Flour
› Almond Meal

MEATS AND PROTEINS

› Bacon/Sausage
› Beef
› Chicken
› Deli Meat
› Eggs
› Fish
› Hot Dogs
› Pork
› Shellfish
› Tofu

DAIRY

› Almond Milk, *unsweetened*
› Cheese
› Coconut Milk, *unsweetened*
› Cottage Cheese
› Cream Cheese
› Greek Yogurt
› Heavy Cream
› Low-Carb Yogurt
› Sour Cream

FATS

› Almond Butter
› Butter
› Flax Meal
› Mayonnaise
› Nuts/Seeds
› Oils
› Natural Peanut Butter
› Salad Dressing
› Ranch Dressing
› Shortening

BEVERAGES

› Black Tea, *decaffeinated*
› Diet Rite® Soda
› Herbal Tea
› Powerade® Zero
› Sparkling Water
› Flavored Water, calorie-free

MISCELLANEOUS

› Agave Nectar
› Chicken Broth
› Cocoa Powder, *unsweetened*
› Chocolate, *unsweetened*
› DaVinci® Gourmet Sugar Free Syrups
› Decaffeinated Instant Coffee
› Herbs/Spices
› Liquid Sucralose
› Liquid Smoke
› Mustard
› Soy Sauce
› Stevia
› Sugar Free Gelatin
› Pure Vanilla Extract
› Vinegar
› Worcestershire Sauce
› Xanthan Gum
› Yeast

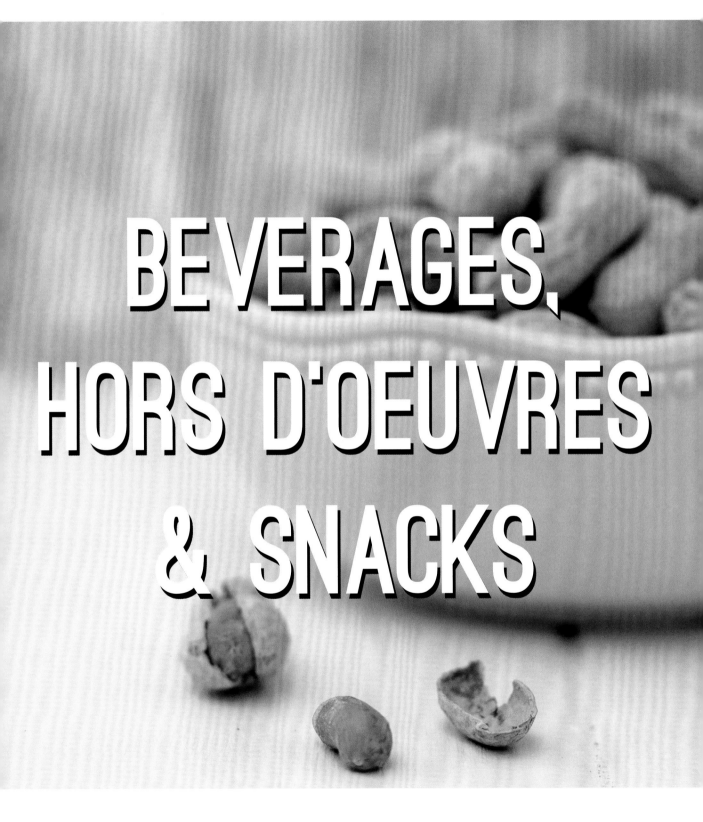

BEVERAGES, HORS D'OEUVRES & SNACKS

small & simple

When we started the Low Glycemic Index Diet, I thought Andria would be drinking nothing but water. Happily, the recipes in this section will prove otherwise. A bit of creativity goes a long way. Although I primarily use sucralose as a sweetener in my beverages, my personal preference would be to use stevia, as it is a more natural product. If you are cooking for someone with less fastidious tastes than I am, try substituting with stevia.

Everyone loves snacks! Admittedly, snacks have been my greatest dilemma. I vividly recall having Andria walk in the door after school and feeling tense because I did not know what she was going to have for a snack. With time, I discovered several allies, the best of which was simply being prepared. Snacks at school on special days posed a unique problem. When all the other mommies were coming to school with sugar laden or carb rich trays, what was I to take? One day I fixed individual, disposable 2 ounce cups on a large tray. In half the cups I had sugar free Jell-O® cubes with two flavors mixed, and the other half I had mixed fresh berries—blueberries, raspberries, and straw-berries. Want to know a little secret? The fruit tray was the first to be emptied! Now that is a mother's true success!

In addition to recipes, I have included a list of simple snack ideas that require little or no cook-ing. Here's to snacking!

SNACK IDEAS

› Hard boiled eggs, carrots, and celery sticks (serve with sea salt)
› Peanuts or mixed nuts of choice
› Yogurt parfaits (layer low carb vanilla yogurt with fresh berries and chopped, toasted pecans)
› Ham and cheese kabobs
› Fresh berries on skewers
› Whole strawberries with Real Whipped Cream (see Index), for dipping
› String cheese
› Pickles
› Olives
› Assorted cheeses
› Veggies and ranch dressing for dipping
› Deli meat and cheese roll-ups
› Sugar Free Jell-O®
› Sugar Free Popsicle®
› Nut butters on celery sticks

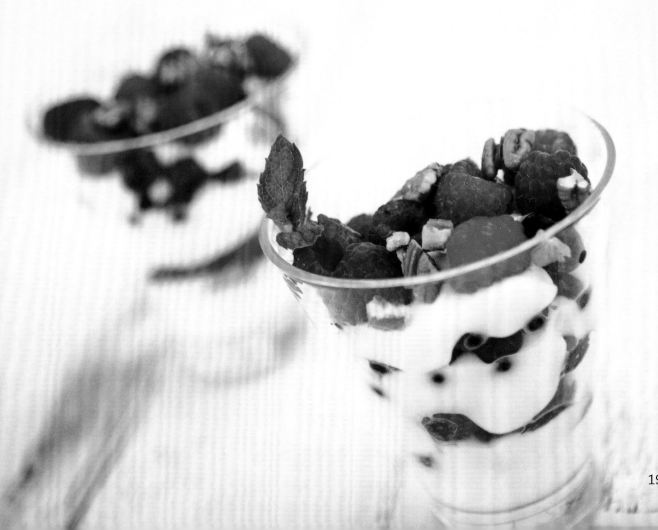

BACON WRAPPED SMOKIES

This is a sure hit at children's parties or school functions!

16 cocktail smokies
8 slices bacon, cut in half

Preheat oven to 400°. Line baking sheet with foil and spray with nonstick cooking spray. Wrap each smokie in half a piece of bacon, securing with a toothpick if necessary.

Place on baking sheet. Bake for 12 minutes. Remove toothpicks. Turn broiler on high and broil for 2 or 3 minutes. Serve immediately.

Makes 16 Servings

TIPS TO TRY

Try shrimp instead of smokies, or cook on the grill instead of in the oven.

NUTRITIONAL FACTS

Serving Size 2 Smokies
Amount per serving:
Calories 304
Total Fat 27.0g
Total Carbohydrate 1.6g
Dietary Fiber 0g
Sugars 1.4g
Protein 13.6g

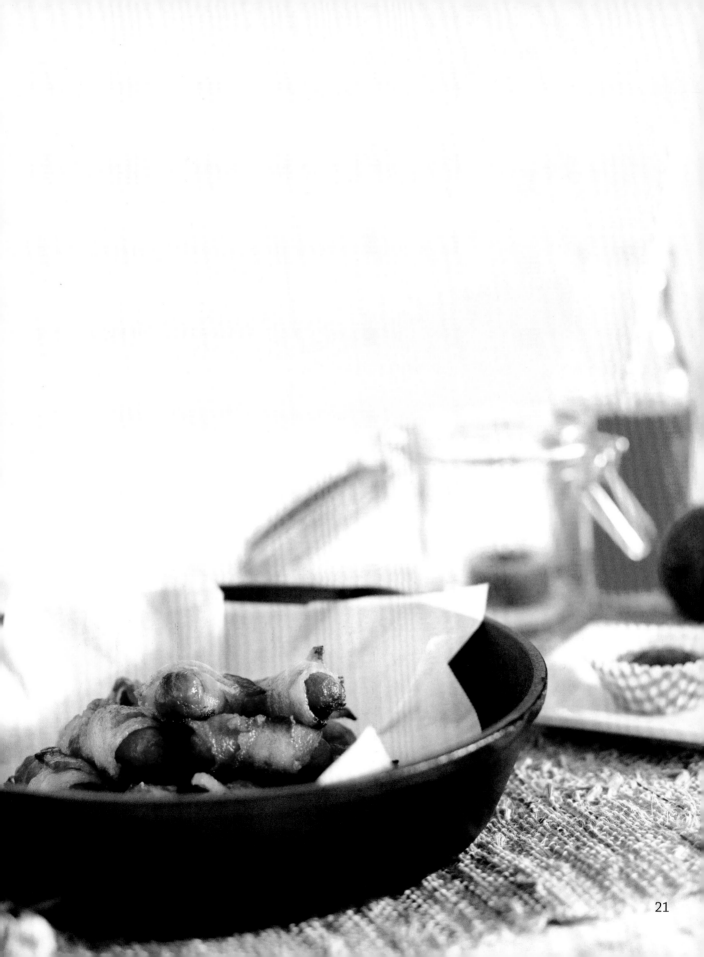

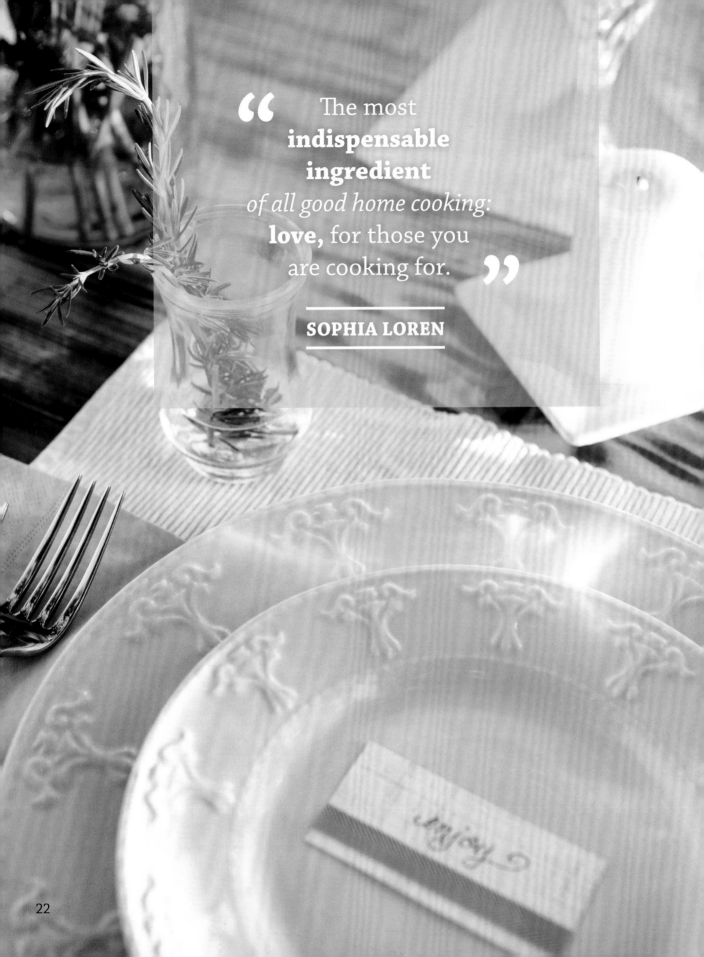

> " The most **indispensable ingredient** *of all good home cooking:* **love,** for those you are cooking for. "
>
> **SOPHIA LOREN**

TACO TORTILLA PINWHEELS

A fun snack for little fingers. Add or subtract herbs and seasonings to fit your personal taste buds.

2 teaspoons Taco Seasoning (see Index)
2 ounces cream cheese, softened
⅛ teaspoon cumin
⅛ teaspoon parsley
Sea salt and freshly ground pepper, to taste
¼-½ cup shredded cheddar cheese
¼ cup Refried Beans (see Index)
Finely chopped onion and green peppers, optional
2 low carb 8" tortillas

Combine all the ingredients (except tortillas) in a mixing bowl, and mix by hand or with mixer. Divide mixture between 2 tortillas and roll up. Wrap tightly in plastic wrap and refrigerate for 2 hours.

With sharp knife, slice each tortilla into 1" pinwheels. Serve with salsa or ranch dressing as a dip.

Makes 2 Servings

Taco Tortilla Pinwheels pictured on pg. 26.

TIPS TO TRY

These pinwheels can also be sliced and served on skewers. Alternate with chunks of colby or cheddar cheese.

NUTRITIONAL FACTS

Serving Size 1 Tortilla
Amount per serving:
Calories 271
Total Fat 14.8g
Total Carbohydrate 19.9g
Dietary Fiber 11g
Sugars 1g
Protein 10.3g

CINNAMON TORTILLA PINWHEELS

A sweet and spicy snack item, cinnamon pinwheels are great for after school or in a lunch box.

1 low carb 8" tortilla
2 tablespoons cream cheese, softened
Pinch of cinnamon
Dash of liquid sucralose or 1 drop of liquid stevia

Combine cream cheese, cinnamon, and sweetener. Mix well.

Spread on tortilla and roll up. Wrap securely in plastic wrap and refrigerate for 2 hours. With very sharp knife, slice into 1" pinwheels. Enjoy!

Makes 2 Servings

TIPS TO TRY

Add any other spices that appeal to you, such as cloves, ginger, allspice, or nutmeg.

NUTRITIONAL FACTS

Serving Size 1/2 Tortilla
Amount per serving:
Calories 142
Total Fat 9.7g
Total Carbohydrate 8.2g
Dietary Fiber 5g
Sugars 1g
Protein 4.2g

CINNAMON TORTILLA CHIPS

Instead of baking, try deep-frying these chips in oil, then sprinkle with cinnamon.

2 low carb 8" tortillas, each cut into 8 triangles
Olive oil or melted butter
Cinnamon

Preheat oven to 250°. Spray tortilla wedges lightly with olive oil or brush with melted butter. Sprinkle with cinnamon.

Place on greased baking sheet. Bake for 1 hour.

Makes 4 Servings

NUTRITIONAL FACTS

Serving Size 4 Chips	
Amount per serving:	
Calories 55	
Total Fat 1.1g	
Total Carbohydrate 7g	
Dietary Fiber 5g	
Sugars 0g	
Protein 2.5g	

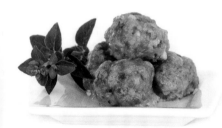 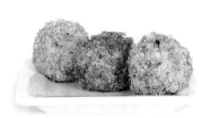 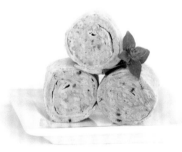

Left to right: *Cheesy Sausage Balls; Mini Cheese Balls; Taco Tortilla Pinwheels.*

MINI CHEESE BALLS

I created this version of my regular cheese ball in my days of snack desperation. Serve with Cheese Snack Crackers (see Index) or alternate with Cheesy Sausage Balls (see Index) on skewers for a fun presentation.

8 ounces shredded colby or cheddar cheese
4 ounces cream cheese, softened
Sprinkle of garlic powder
¼ teaspoon sea salt
2 tablespoons salad dressing
¼ cup pecans, ground
¼ cup fried bacon, crumbled

Mix first 5 ingredients in mixer. Shape into 1" balls. Roll half the balls in ground pecans, and half in bacon pieces.

If serving on skewers, refrigerate until firm before threading skewers. Chill before serving.

Makes 24 Servings

TIPS TO TRY

To grind pecans, pulse in mini chopper for 15 seconds.

NUTRITIONAL FACTS

Serving Size 1 Cheese Ball

Amount per serving:

Calories 73

Total Fat 6.5g

Total Carbohydrate 0.7g

Dietary Fiber 0g

Sugars 0g

Protein 3.2g

CHEESY SAUSAGE BALLS

1 pound sausage, fried
2 cups shredded cheddar cheese
½ cup fine bread crumbs (see Index for Almond Meal Dinner Rolls and Bread Crumbs)
¼ cup finely minced onion
¼ teaspoon garlic salt

Preheat oven to 375°. Combine all ingredients and mix well. Form into 1" balls and place on greased baking pan.

Bake for 15 minutes.

Makes 22 Servings

Cheesy Sausage Balls pictured on pg. 26.

TIPS TO TRY

Try these on skewers with cheese chunks for a fun appetizer, or serve with party picks.

NUTRITIONAL FACTS

Serving Size 1 Sausage Ball
Amount per serving:
Calories 132
Total Fat 11.3g
Total Carbohydrate 1.3g
Dietary Fiber 0g
Sugars 0g
Protein 6.2g

CHEESE SNACK CRACKERS

Pull out your cookie cutters and get creative! Homemade crackers are lots of fun.

¾ cup shredded colby or cheddar cheese
6 tablespoons almond meal
Dash of paprika
½ teaspoon sea salt
2 tablespoons cold butter, cubed
1-2 tablespoons heavy whipping cream

Preheat oven to 350°. Place the cheese, almond meal, paprika, and salt in food processor; process until blended. Add butter. Pulse until butter is the size of peas. Continue pulsing, adding just enough cream to form moist crumbs.

Using additional almond meal to lightly dust surface, roll dough to 1/8" thickness. Cut with a 2" cookie cutter, or cut into 10 squares with pizza cutter.

Place on baking sheet. Bake for 13-17 minutes or until golden. Store in airtight container.

Makes 10 Servings

NUTRITIONAL FACTS

Serving Size 1 Cracker

Amount per serving:

Calories 79

Total Fat 7.3g

Total Carbohydrate 1.0g

Dietary Fiber 0g

Sugars 0g

Protein 2.8g

HUMMUS

This is, hands down, the best hummus. I start with dried chickpeas and cook my own beans, using the Master Bean Method (see Index). You can also use canned chickpeas, more commonly known as garbanzo beans. The day I first mixed the hummus I simply couldn't stop eating it!

Make your own tahini paste:
6 tablespoons sesame seeds
4 tablespoons water
1 teaspoon olive oil
2 teaspoons lemon juice

Preheat oven to 350°. Spread sesame seeds on baking sheet and toast for 6-8 minutes. Watch closely—do not brown. Cool. Place in blender or food processor with other ingredients and blend until smooth. Store tahini in refrigerator for up to several weeks.

Makes 1/3 Cup

2 cups garbanzo beans (drain, but save 2 tablespoons liquid)
1 teaspoon sea salt
2 cloves garlic
⅓ cup tahini paste (see above)
7-8 tablespoons lemon juice (fresh, if possible)
2 tablespoons liquid from drained beans
Olive oil
4-8 drops Tabasco® sauce
Crudités for dipping: celery sticks, baby carrots, broccoli, and bell peppers

Blend first 6 ingredients in blender until smooth. (Adjust salt and garlic to suit your personal taste.)

Before serving, spritz with olive oil and Tabasco®. Serve with crudités.

Makes 32 Servings

TIPS TO TRY

Create a Mediterranean wrap: spread hummus on low carb tortilla; add turkey, cheese of choice, and olives; fold and roll!

NUTRITIONAL FACTS

Serving Size 1 Tablespoon
Amount per serving:
Calories 41
Total Fat 2.7g
Total Carbohydrate 3.4g
Dietary Fiber 1g
Sugars 0g
Protein 1.4g

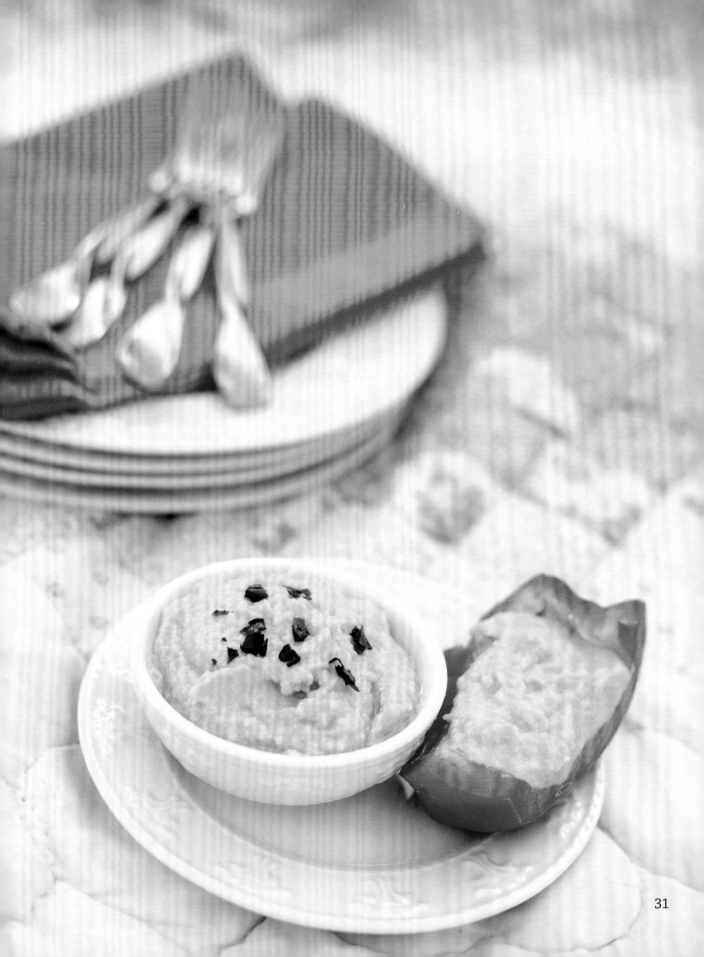

31

RANCH PECAN SNACKS

Living in the South, we have the advantage of buying locally grown pecans. The idea for this recipe was born from the more traditional ranch pretzel snack mix that my family practically inhales.

¼ cup olive oil
¼ teaspoon dill weed, optional
1 tablespoon ranch dressing mix
⅛ teaspoon garlic salt
¼ teaspoon lemon pepper
2 cups raw pecan halves

Preheat oven to 250°. In medium sized bowl, combine first 5 ingredients and whisk with fork. Add pecans, stirring to coat. Spread on greased baking sheet.

Toast in oven for 30 minutes, stirring after 15 minutes. Cool. Divide into 1/4 cup servings.

Makes 8 Servings

NUTRITIONAL FACTS

Serving Size 1/4 Cup

Amount per serving:

Calories 234

Total Fat 24.6g

Total Carbohydrate 4.2g

Dietary Fiber 2g

Sugars 1g

Protein 2.3g

TOASTED NUT MIX

2 tablespoons butter, melted
¼ teaspoon liquid stevia
Dash of cinnamon
Dash of nutmeg
1½ cups roasted peanuts
1 cup roasted pumpkin seeds

Preheat oven to 300°. In small bowl, mix all ingredients with a fork.

Spread on baking sheet and toast for 1 hour, stirring every 15 minutes. Cool, then divide into individual snack bags with 2 tablespoons in each bag. May be stored in freezer.

Makes 20 Servings

NUTRITIONAL FACTS

Serving Size 2 Tablespoons	
Amount per serving:	
Calories 108	
Total Fat 9.7g	
Total Carbohydrate 2.5g	
Dietary Fiber 1g	
Sugars 1g	
Protein 4.8g	

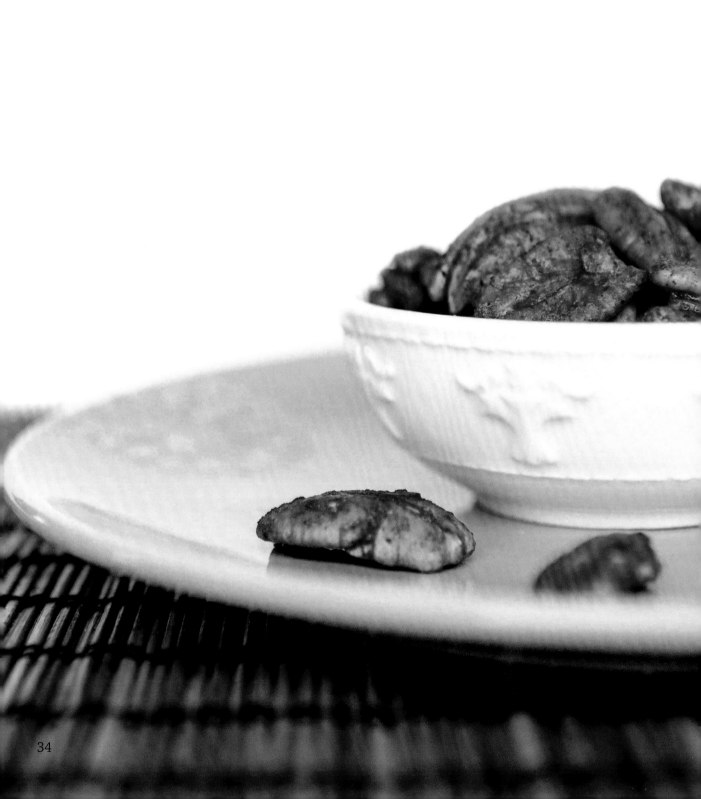

SPICED PECANS

1 egg white
2 tablespoons DaVinci® Pancake Sugar Free Syrup (or flavor of your choice)
2 cups raw pecan halves
2 teaspoons chili powder
1 teaspoon cinnamon
1 teaspoon sea salt
¼ teaspoon cayenne pepper, optional

Preheat oven to 300°. In large bowl, lightly whisk egg white for 15-20 seconds, then whisk in syrup until blended. Toss pecans into mixture and stir to coat evenly. Add remaining ingredients.

Transfer pecans to parchment lined baking sheet. Bake at 300° for 25 minutes, until pecans are browned and mixture is dry. Cool and break into pieces for serving.

Makes 16 Servings

TIPS TO TRY

Measure these pecans out in 2 tablespoon amounts and package individually for a quick, take-along snack.

NUTRITIONAL FACTS

Serving Size 2 Tablespoons	
Amount per serving:	
Calories 87	
Total Fat 8.9g	
Total Carbohydrate 1.7g	
Dietary Fiber 1g	
Sugars 1g	
Protein 1.4g	

CREAM FILLED STRAWBERRIES

1 ounce cream cheese, softened
¼ cup Real Whipped Cream (see Index)
6 strawberries, washed and hulled

Beat cream cheese until smooth and creamy. Gently add Real Whipped Cream.

Cut small point off top and bottom of strawberries. Setting the berry upright, cut an "X" partway through the berry, pulling all 4 pieces slightly apart to create a "well" in the middle of the berry. Use decorating bag to fill center with approximately 1 tablespoon filling. Refrigerate.

Makes 6 Servings

NUTRITIONAL FACTS

Serving Size 1 Strawberry
Amount per serving:
Calories 43
Total Fat 4.1g
Total Carbohydrate 1.4g
Dietary Fiber 0g
Sugars 1g
Protein 0.5g

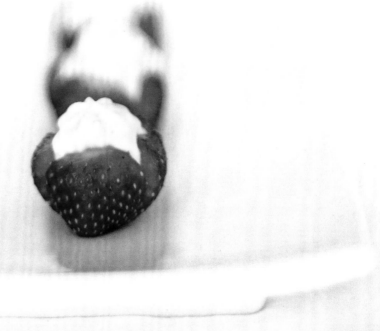

an apple a day...

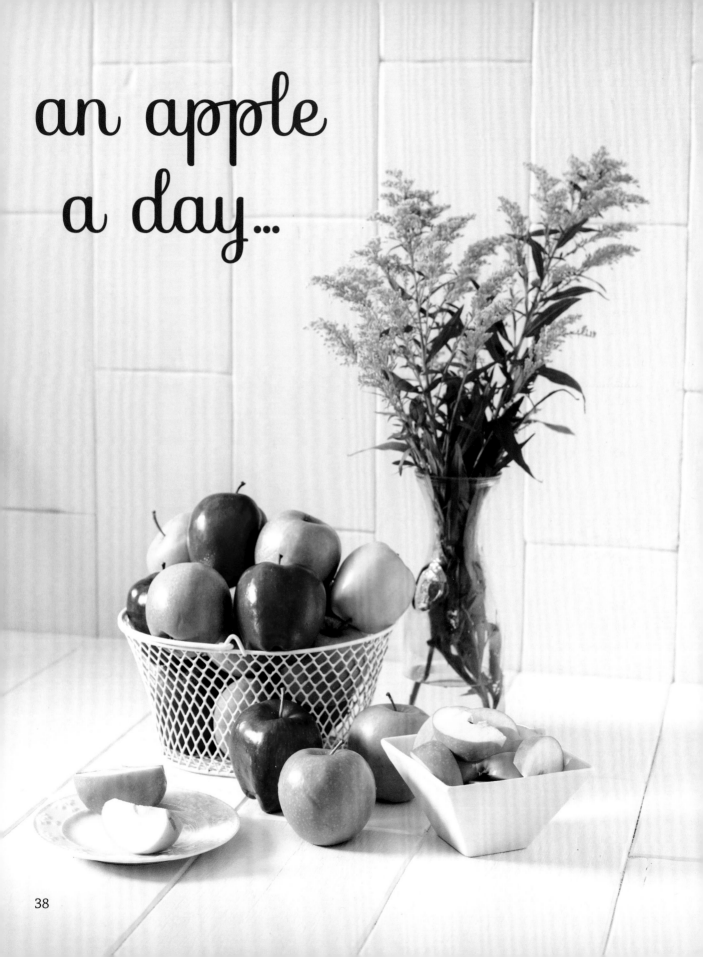

QUESADILLA APPLE PIE
Yummy, yummy! This piece of Americana is as fun to fix as it is to eat.

2 teaspoons butter
½ apple, thinly sliced
Sprinkle of cinnamon
Sprinkle of nutmeg
1 tablespoon cream cheese, softened
1 low carb 8" tortilla

In small skillet, melt butter. Add apples and spices. Fry until apples are soft and a bit mushy. Spread softened cream cheese on tortilla. Pour apple mixture on 1/2 of tortilla.

Fold tortilla gently and place on preheated quesadilla maker. Fry until edges of tortilla are brown and slightly crisp. Serve warm with Real Whipped Cream (see Index).

Makes 2 Servings

Because the carb amount on this treat is a bit higher than some other desserts, it takes a little planning to incorporate. I use it on days when Andria's other carbs are lower than normal, or on special occasions when the rest of the family is enjoying some treat forbidden to the low glycemic diet.

> ***Core half an apple—fill center with 1 teaspoon natural peanut butter.***

Nutritional Facts for these recipes can be found on page 187.

PEANUT BUTTER
¼ cup low carb vanilla yogurt
1 tablespoon creamy natural peanut butter

In small bowl, combine yogurt and peanut butter with spoon. Serve with apple slices.
Makes 1 Serving

CARAMEL
¼ cup Real Whipped Cream (see Index)
½ teaspoon DaVinci® Caramel Sugar Free Syrup
½ teaspoon pure vanilla extract

Blend all ingredients with spoon. Serve with apple slices. **Makes 1 Serving**

APPLE CHIPS
Apple chips are a big hit at our house. Divide into snack bags with half an apple in each bag, and store in the freezer.

1 apple

Preheat oven to 250°. Spray wire rack with non-stick cooking spray and place on baking sheet. Core and quarter apple, then slice as thinly as possible, preferably paper-thin. Spread apple slices on wire rack and sprinkle with cinnamon. Bake for 2½ hours. Cool completely before packaging.

Makes 2 Servings

If you don't have wire racks (I use the type for cooling cookies), placing the apple directly on the greased baking sheet will work as well.

STRAWBERRY MILKSHAKE

2 whole strawberries, washed and hulled
3 ice cubes
½ cup Real Whipped Cream (see Index)
2–3 tablespoons cold water
¼ teaspoon clear imitation vanilla flavoring

Place all ingredients in blender and blend on high until smooth. Serve in a tall glass with additional Real Whipped Cream for garnish.

Makes 1 Serving

TIPS TO TRY

For many milkshake days, I couldn't concoct something Andria would drink. It seemed the blender action with the heavy whipping cream caused it to curdle. One day I used leftover Real Whipped Cream. Presto! It looked like a real milkshake, and Andria drained the cup. Be sure to whip the cream first.

NUTRITIONAL FACTS

Serving Size 8 Ounces
Amount per serving:
Calories 285
Total Fat 29.4g
Total Carbohydrate 5.1g
Dietary Fiber 0g
Sugars 1g
Protein 1.8g

a la yum...

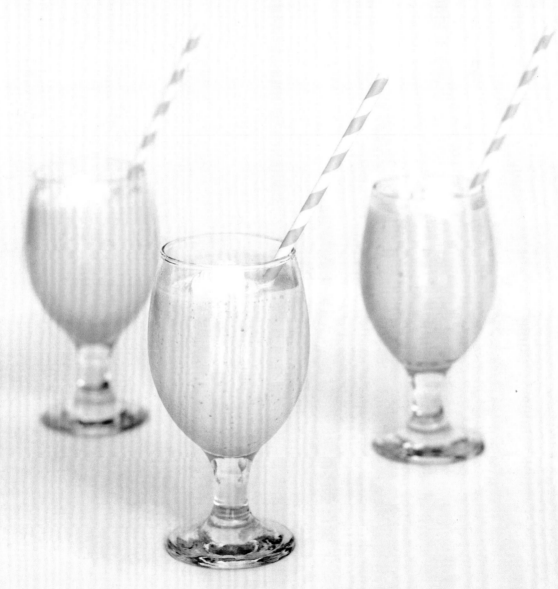

RASPBERRY SMOOTHIE

2 tablespoons raspberries
¼ cup low carb vanilla yogurt
4 ice cubes
2-3 tablespoons cold water

Combine all ingredients in blender and pulse until thickened and smooth. Pour into tall glass and serve. Garnish with Real Whipped Cream (see Index), if desired.

Makes 1 Serving

NUTRITIONAL FACTS

Serving Size 8 Ounces
Amount per serving:
Calories 28
Total Fat 0.8g
Total Carbohydrate 3.1g
Dietary Fiber 1g
Sugars 2g
Protein 2.9g

RASPBERRY SWEET TEA

Sweet tea is a staple at our house. We drink it every day throughout the summertime, and always serve it for Sunday dinner. To make unflavored sweet tea, follow instructions below, simply omitting the raspberry syrup. You can also experiment with any other flavored syrup that suits your fancy.

1 cup water
1 family size decaf tea bag
10 drops liquid sucralose
1 teaspoon DaVinci® Raspberry Sugar Free Syrup
Additional water and ice

Starting with fresh, cold water, bring water to a boil. Pour over tea bag, and brew 5 minutes.

Fill 1 quart pitcher 1/4 full of ice cubes; add sucralose. Pour hot tea over ice and stir briskly. Add raspberry syrup, then additional water and ice to make 1 quart. Serve over ice.

Makes 4 Servings

NUTRITIONAL FACTS

*This is considered a **free food** as the carbs are low enough to remain uncalculated.*

RASPBERRY LEMONADE

Rosy color over clinking ice cubes makes this a party must-have. Refreshing and tangy, the classic lemonade gets a lovely twist of raspberry. This drink is eye catching and delicious!

2 lemons
2 teaspoons DaVinci® Raspberry Sugar Free Syrup
10 drops liquid sucralose
Ice and water to make 1 quart
Additional lemon slices for garnish

Squeeze juice from lemons, straining out seeds. Mix all ingredients in 1 quart pitcher. Adjust sweetener to suit your taste.

Makes 4 Servings

NUTRITIONAL FACTS

Serving Size 8 Ounces
Amount per serving:
Calories 6
Total Fat 0.1g
Total Carbohydrate 1.7g
Dietary Fiber 0g
Sugars 1g
Protein 0.1g

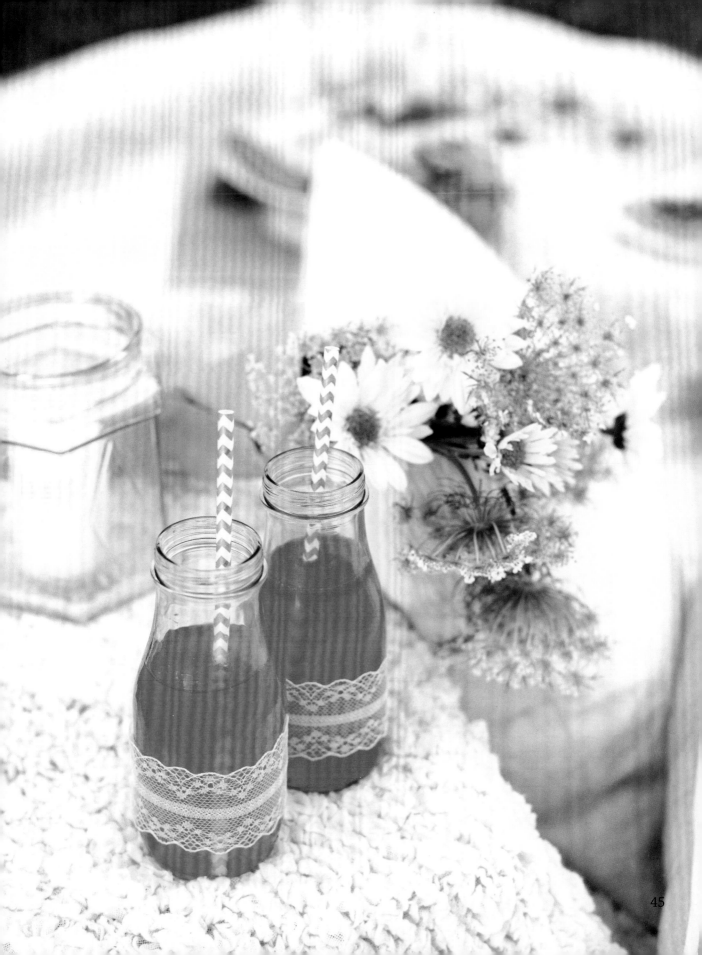

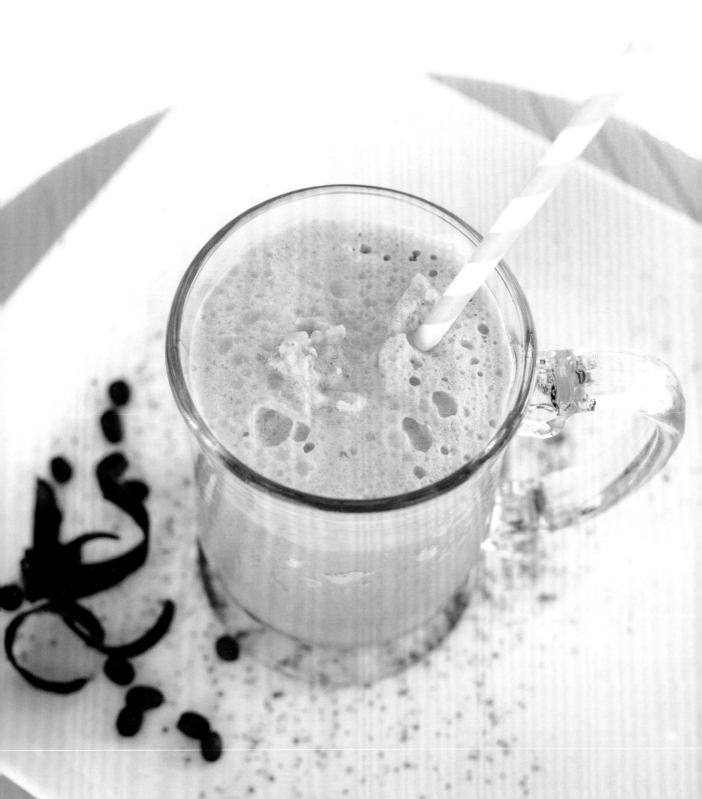

FROSTY MOCHACCINO

Our family adores coffee drinks. Swap the chocolate syrup for caramel, or use cocoa powder and a pinch of sweetener. Sit in the sunshine as you sip!

½ cup Real Whipped Cream (see Index)
1 teaspoon DaVinci® Chocolate Sugar Free Syrup
1 teaspoon cocoa
3 drops liquid sucralose
½ teaspoon decaf instant coffee
5 ice cubes
6 tablespoons cold water
Additional Real Whipped Cream (see Index) and cocoa for garnish

Combine first 7 ingredients in blender and pulse until ice is blended. Pour into a tall glass mug; garnish, and serve immediately.

Makes 1 Serving

NUTRITIONAL FACTS

Serving Size 8 Ounces

Amount per serving:

Calories 284

Total Fat 29.5g

Total Carbohydrate 4.8g

Dietary Fiber 1g

Sugars 0g

Protein 2.1g

COZY HOT COCOA

I knew there had to be a way to make hot cocoa for Andria. With butter, cream, and cocoa, certainly I could create something comforting. Here it is—grab your mug and a cinnamon stick!

2 teaspoons butter
1½ cups water
1 tablespoon cocoa
2 teaspoons pure vanilla extract
Pinch of sea salt
½ cup heavy whipping cream
8 drops liquid sucralose
Cinnamon to taste, optional

In heavy saucepan, melt butter. Add cocoa, water, vanilla, and salt. Bring to a boil and simmer for 3 minutes, stirring constantly. Add sucralose and cream. When well heated, pour into mugs and serve.

Makes 2 Servings

TIPS TO TRY

Instead of the traditional marshmallows, garnish with Real Whipped Cream (see Index) and dust with cinnamon or cocoa.

NUTRITIONAL FACTS

Serving Size 8 Ounces
Amount per serving:
Calories 257
Total Fat 26.2g
Total Carbohydrate 3.8g
Dietary Fiber 1g
Sugars 1g
Protein 1.8g

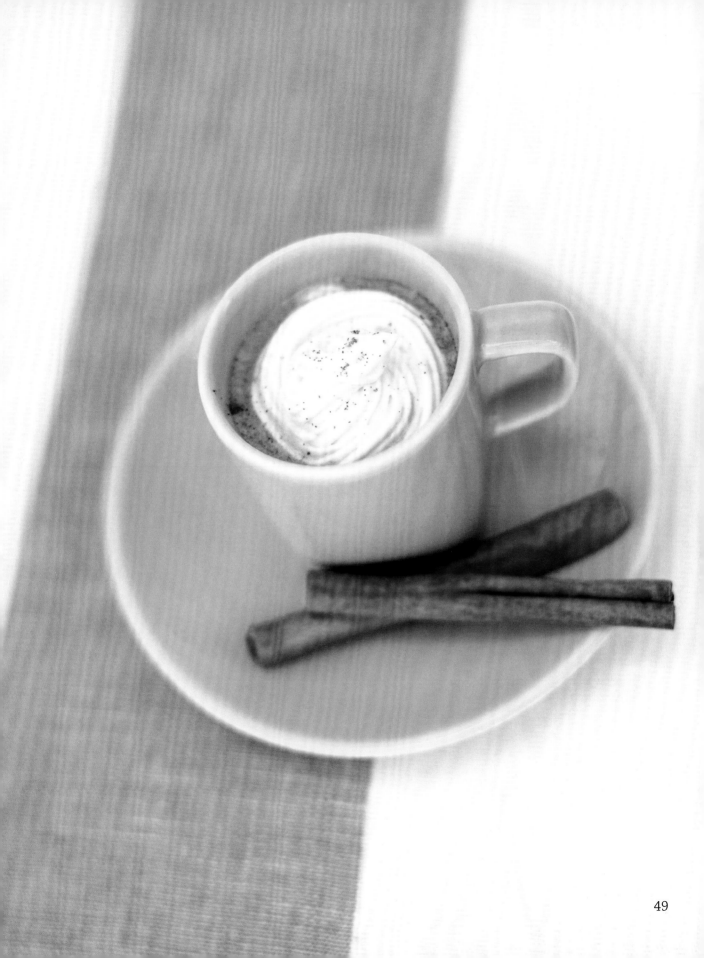

49

FOR SPECIAL DAYS

» Diet Rite® Soda

» Sugar Free Popsicles®

» Breyer's® Low Carb Vanilla Ice Cream

» Sugar Free Gum

» Ice Cream Float with Diet Rite® Soda and Low Carb Ice Cream

» Sugar Free Refrigerated Jell-O® Cups

EATING ON THE GO

SUBWAY® Oven roasted chicken breast and a side of apple slices (with salad, or order the chicken only as a side with melted cheese on top).

MCDONALDS® Order the premium grilled chicken breast with melted cheese and no bun. Ask for ranch on the side to use for dipping.

CHICK-FIL-A® Grilled chicken nuggets with ranch on the side.

DINE-IN RESTAURANTS Stick with grilled chicken if possible. There are less chances of additives compared to ground beef. Salad and fruit bars are great!

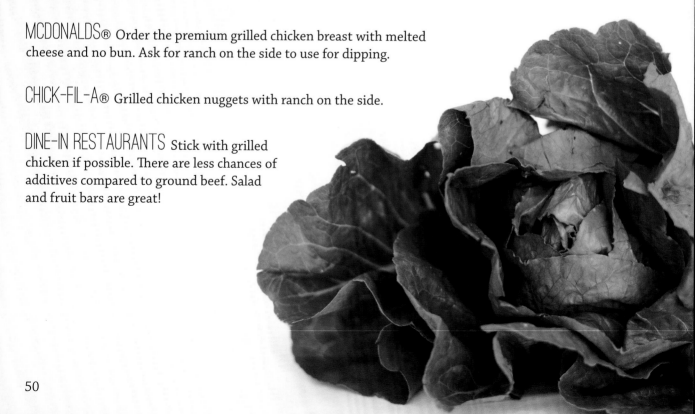

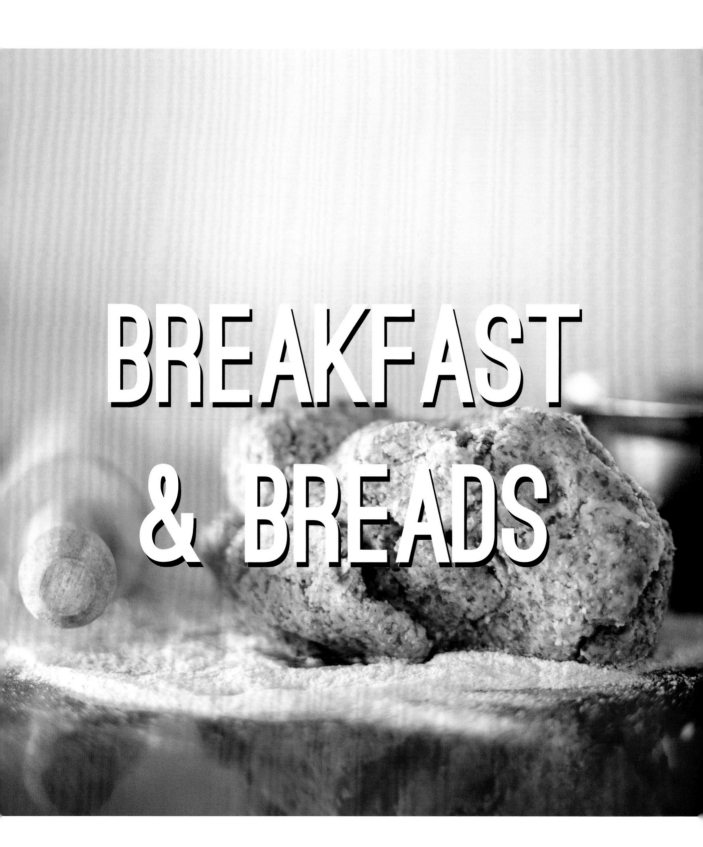

BREAKFAST
& BREADS

rise and shine

For a morning eye-opener on the low glyce-mic diet, zero in on the wonderful simplicity of the egg! Unfortunately for us, eggs were not among the foods Andria enjoyed. With time, we have made progress, but the Almond Meal Pancakes have been our mainstay since the beginning of the diet. Breakfast needs to be un-complicated, yet nutritious and filling, especially if you are sending a son or daughter off for a day of school. I had the advantage of being at home during the day, so I would make the pancakes at any time except in the morning's mad rush, then freeze them. This allowed us to develop a very comfortable and workable morning routine.

In addition to the recipes I have included here, think meat on the side for breakfast. Sausage,

bacon, ham.... We make our own sausage every winter, so breakfast often included a grilled sausage patty with the pancake. Again, almost any meat can be grilled ahead of time and frozen in individual portions.

The breads have been more difficult. I have tried and retried recipes, and so far the bread and tortillas I buy have passed the taste and low carb test better than anything I have been able to make, with the exception of the Almond Meal Dinner Rolls.

Nothing says love like a *good morning* breakfast!

BACON, EGG & CHEESE BREAKFAST SANDWICH

1 low carb flatbread or 1 slice low carb bread of choice
2 teaspoons sour cream or butter
**1 egg, scrambled, with sea salt and freshly ground pepper
to taste**
1 tablespoon fried bacon, crumbled
3 tablespoons shredded cheddar cheese

Place flatbread in toaster and toast lightly. Spread with sour
cream or butter. Place scrambled egg on top and add bacon and
cheese.

Microwave for 12 seconds to melt cheese.

Makes 1 Serving

NUTRITIONAL FACTS

Serving Size 1 Sandwich
Amount per serving:
Calories 307
Total Fat 19.9g
Total Carbohydrate 16g
Dietary Fiber 7g
Sugars 1g
Protein 21.7g

SUNRISE OMELETS

Basic omelet:

2 eggs
1 tablespoon water
Sea salt and freshly ground pepper, to taste

Choose your filling (on right).

In small bowl, lightly whisk eggs, water, salt, and pepper with fork.

Spray 8" nonstick skillet and place on burner. Preheat slightly with burner turned to medium-high. Pour egg mixture into skillet.

As egg fries, lift outer edges gently with spatula to allow unfried sections to flow to outside. When set, place fillings of choice in center of omelet and sprinkle with salt and pepper.

With spatula, fold outside third of omelet over fillings in center. Repeat with other side. As the omelet is flipped onto serving plate, flip upside down to make third fold complete.

Remove from heat and serve immediately.

Makes 1 Serving

Choose your fillings:

Vegetarian:
2 tablespoons (each): mushrooms, peppers, and onions, sautéed
2 tablespoons shredded cheese of choice
Mediterranean:
1 tablespoon black olives
Fresh basil, minced
1 tablespoon diced tomatoes
2 tablespoons shredded mozzarella cheese
Sausage and feta:
2 tablespoons fried sausage
2 tablespoons feta cheese
3 leaves baby spinach, chopped
Southwest:
2 tablespoons black beans, slightly mashed
1 tablespoon salsa
2 tablespoons shredded colby-jack cheese
Sprinkle of cilantro

NUTRITIONAL FACTS *

Serving Size 1 Omelet
Amount per serving:
Calories 144
Total Fat 9.5g
Total Carbohydrate 0.7g
Dietary Fiber 0g
Sugars 0g
Protein 12.6g

Nutrition Facts are for the Basic Omelet. The nutrition information for the filling options can be found on page 187.

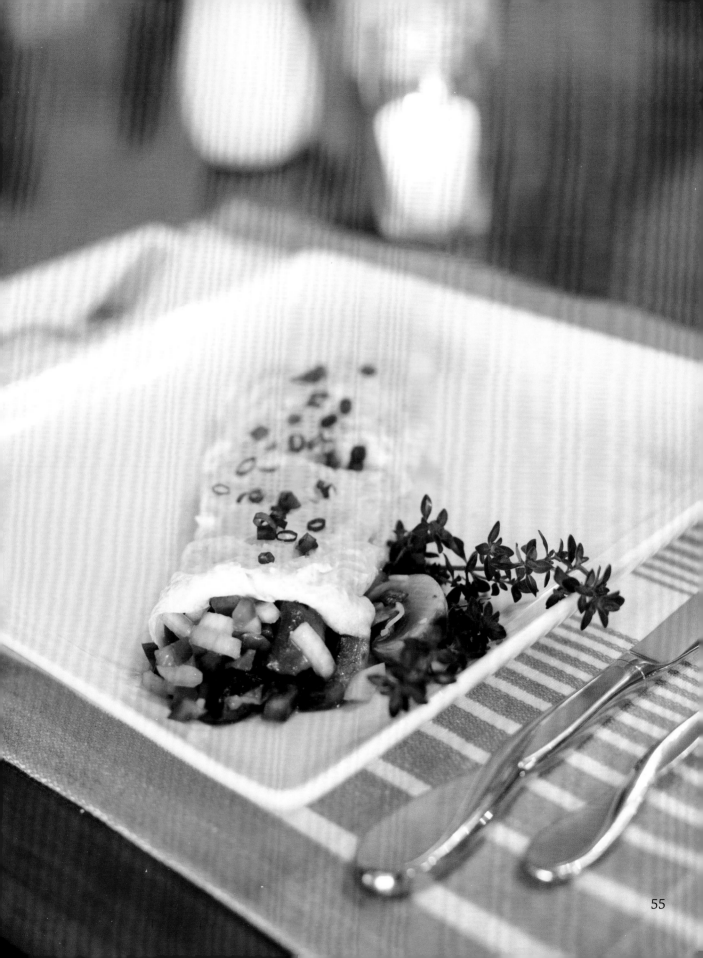

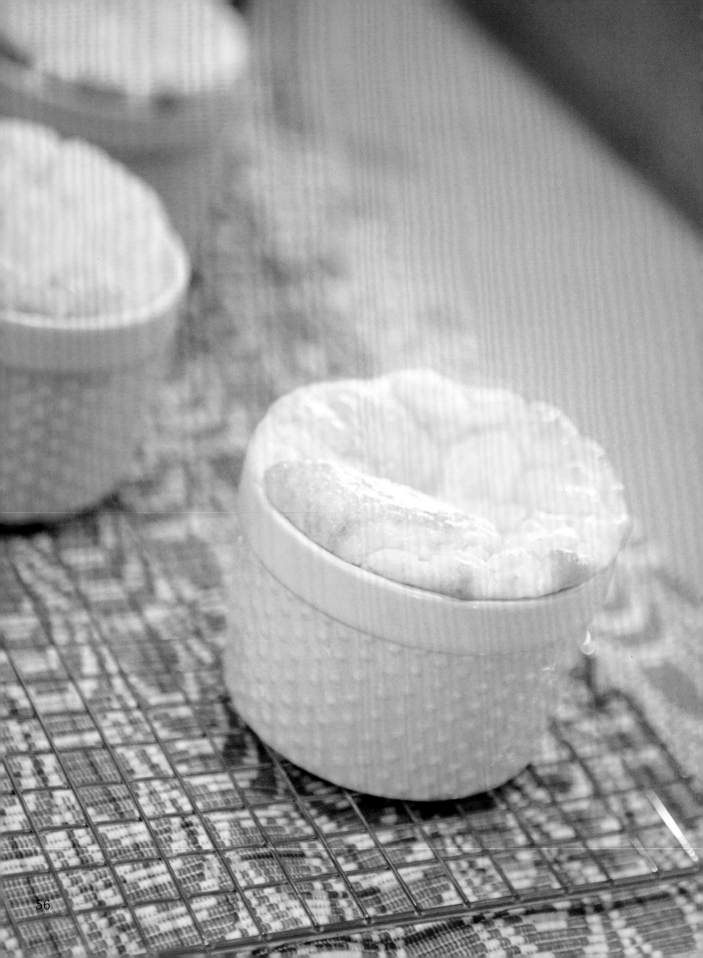

MINI QUICHE

Whip up some handheld fun for breakfast. It's easy to sneak in some veggies as well.

2 eggs
½ cup heavy whipping cream, mixed with ¼ cup water
2 ounces cream cheese, softened
Sea salt and freshly ground pepper, to taste
2 tablespoons fried bacon, crumbled
4 tablespoons shredded cheddar cheese

Preheat oven to 375°. In small bowl, whisk eggs, cream, cream cheese, salt, and pepper. Fold in bacon and cheese.

Pour into silicone baking cups or well greased muffin pan, filling each one 3/4 full. Bake for 20 minutes or until toothpick inserted in center comes out clean. Garnish with shredded cheese.

Makes 6 Servings

TIPS TO TRY

Try adding sautéed mushrooms, onions, broccoli, or bell peppers for extra flavor.

NUTRITIONAL FACTS

Serving Size 1 Quiche
Amount per serving:
Calories 158
Total Fat 14.9g
Total Carbohydrate 1.2g
Dietary Fiber 0g
Sugars 0g
Protein 5.2g

BREAKFAST EMPANADAS

Frying a low carb tortilla greatly enhances the flavor. This quick breakfast is truly delicious.

2 low carb 8" tortillas
2 eggs, scrambled, with sea salt and freshly ground pepper
to taste
¼ cup fried bacon, crumbled or fried sausage
¼ cup shredded cheddar cheese
butter, softened

Warm tortillas in microwave. Spread both sides with butter. Fill with eggs, meat of your choice, and cheese. Wrap securely, folding both ends in.

Using skillet on stove top, fry empanada until lightly browned and slightly crisp. Flip and fry other side.

Makes 2 Servings

TIPS TO TRY

Breakfast burritos are also fast and easy. Using the ingredients listed, fill tortilla, give it a wrap and a roll, and there's your breakfast to-go.

NUTRITIONAL FACTS

Serving Size 1 Wrap	
Amount per serving:	
Calories 307	
Total Fat 16.5g	
Total Carbohydrate 14.8g	
Dietary Fiber 9g	
Sugars 0g	
Protein 20.6g	

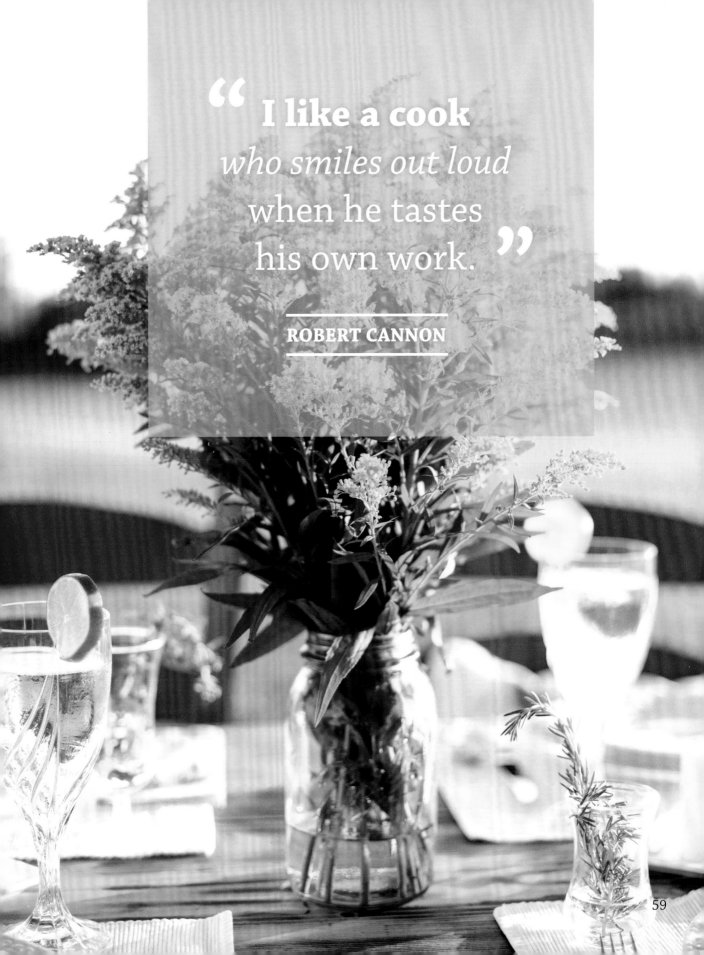

> ❝ **I like a cook**
> *who smiles out loud*
> when he tastes
> his own work. ❞
>
> ──────────
> **ROBERT CANNON**
> ──────────

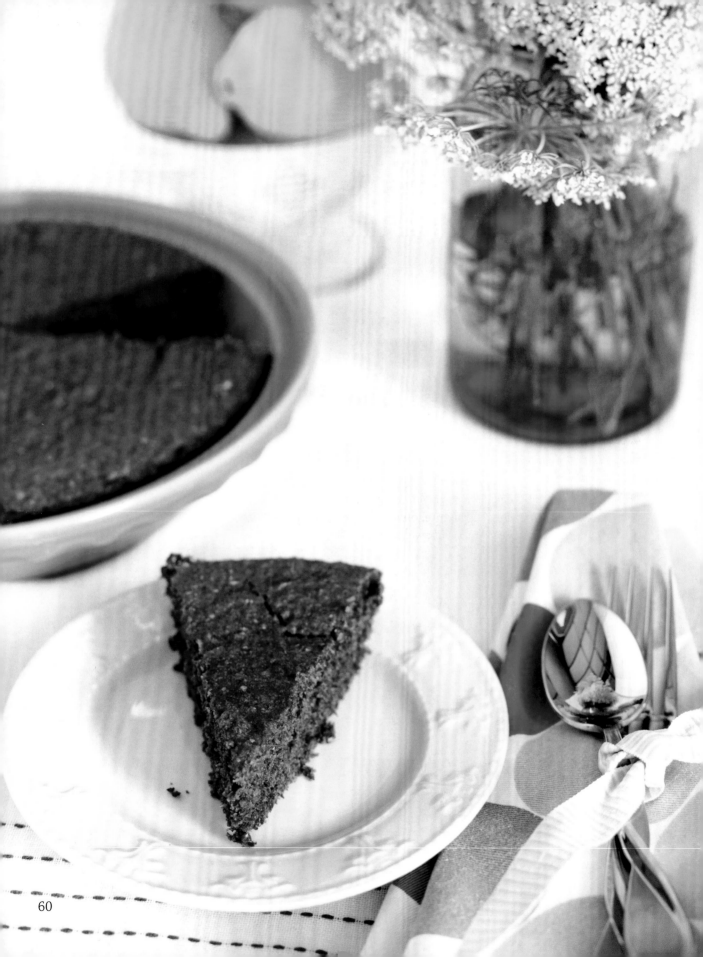

COFFEE GINGERBREAD CAKE

Aromatic and spicy, gingerbread cake will wake the household to cheer as it bakes. The almond meal packs a "stick to your ribs" appeal.

½ cup boiling water
2 tablespoons instant decaf coffee
2 eggs
1 egg white
¼ cup olive oil
⅛ teaspoon liquid stevia
1 tablespoon DaVinci® Pancake Sugar Free Syrup
2½ cups almond meal
½ teaspoon sea salt
1 teaspoon baking soda
1 teaspoon cinnamon
¼ teaspoon cloves
⅛ teaspoon ginger

Preheat oven to 350°. Dissolve coffee in boiling water. In mixer bowl, combine coffee, eggs, egg white, olive oil, stevia, and pancake syrup. Add dry ingredients. Mix well.

Pour into greased 9" round baking pan. Bake for 30 minutes.

Serve warm with a dollop of Real Whipped Cream (see Index), low carb yogurt, or DaVinci® Pancake Sugar Free Syrup.

Makes 10 Servings

TIPS TO TRY

Cut unused cake into individual servings; wrap and freeze the day it is baked. To serve, defrost and warm in microwave.

NUTRITIONAL FACTS

Serving Size 1 Slice	
Amount per serving:	
Calories 204	
Total Fat 18.1g	
Total Carbohydrate 6.1g	
Dietary Fiber 3g	
Sugars 1g	
Protein 6.8g	

ALMOND MEAL PANCAKES

Here is Andria's favorite breakfast food. She ate these pancakes literally every morning for months on end. Served with natural peanut butter and DaVinci® Pancake Sugar Free Syrup, it was a lifesaver for me as well.

2½ cups almond meal
½ cup sprouted wheat flour
½ cup heavy whipping cream
8 eggs
½ cup butter, melted
12 drops liquid stevia
1 tablespoon pure vanilla extract
1 teaspoon baking soda
Pinch of sea salt
¼ cup water

Combine all ingredients and mix well.

Heat griddle and spray with nonstick cooking spray or grease with butter. Drop by 1/4 cupfuls and spread out slightly with back of spoon to flatten. Cook until pancakes are golden and set, about 2 minutes on each side.

Makes 16 Servings

TIPS TO TRY

I made a batch of pancakes every 2 weeks to save time in the mornings. When fried, spread single layer of pancakes on baking sheet and freeze for 1 hour. Stack pancakes and store in gallon size Ziploc® bags in freezer. In the morning, pop a pancake in the microwave for 15 seconds, then toast in toaster. Win-win all the way around, as the almond meal packs a huge protein punch!

NUTRITIONAL FACTS

Serving Size 1 Pancake	
Amount per serving:	
Calories 225	
Total Fat 19.8g	
Total Carbohydrate 6.5g	
Dietary Fiber 1g	
Sugars 1g	
Protein 7.6g	

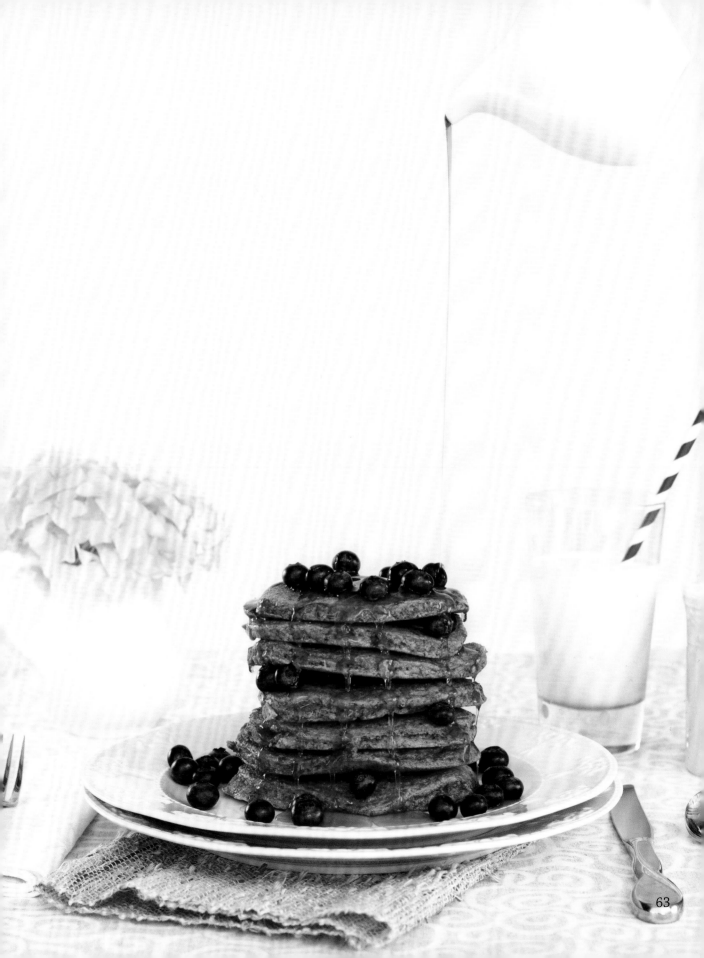

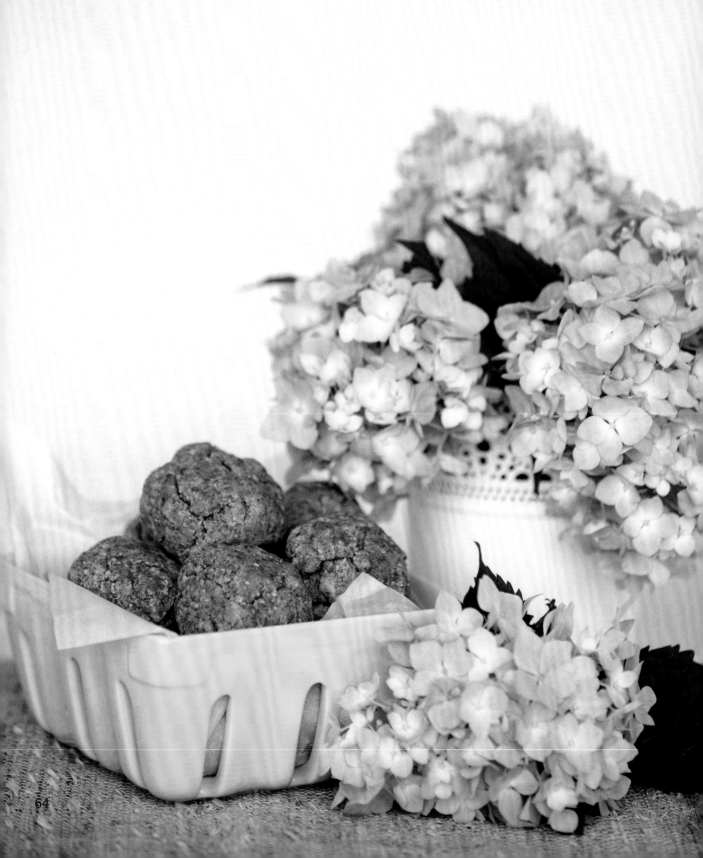

ALMOND MEAL DINNER ROLLS & BREAD CRUMBS

I lost track of how often I tried and retried this recipe. The rolls simply wouldn't rise. A friend gave me invaluable insight on the entire yeast dilemma when she told me that yeast needs some kind of sugar in order to be activated. That was when I tried agave nectar, and there I had my recipe! Try these rolls toasted or microwaved with shredded cheese or natural peanut butter for a quick snack. Surprisingly, my main use for them is as bread crumbs or breading in my other recipes. I keep a Ziploc® bag in the freezer and pull 1 or 2 out as needed.

¾ cup warm water (110°-115°)
2 tablespoons yeast
1 teaspoon agave nectar
2 eggs
½ tablespoon vinegar
¼ cup shortening
1½ teaspoons sea salt
⅛ teaspoon powdered stevia
½ cup sprouted wheat flour
2 tablespoons ground flax seed
1½ tablespoons xanthan gum
4½ cups almond meal

In small bowl, combine warm water, yeast, and agave nectar. Allow yeast to rise for 10 minutes.

Place remaining ingredients (except almond meal) in mixer and mix well. Add yeast mixture. Working dough by hand, or in large stand mixer bowl with dough attachment, gradually add almond meal, 1/2 cup at a time.

Cover with plastic wrap or a light cloth and let rise in a warm place for 2 hours. Punch down and let rise for another 1½ hours.

Form into 17 equal sized dinner rolls and place on lightly greased baking sheet. Cover and let rise for another 2 hours.

Preheat oven to 350°. Bake for 15-20 minutes or until bottom of rolls appear dry.

Makes 17 Servings

TIPS TO TRY

To make fine, dry bread crumbs, place 1 roll in mini food chopper and pulse. 1 roll = 1/4 cup crumbs = 7 grams carbs. Also make crumbs from any of the low carb breads you generally use. Simply calculate the amount of carbs in 1 slice, pulse into crumbs, then measure the finished amount to figure the final carbs.

NUTRITIONAL FACTS

Serving Size 1 Roll
Amount per serving:
Calories 202
Total Fat 16.6g
Total Carbohydrate 9.3g
Dietary Fiber 5g
Sugars 1g
Protein 7.3g

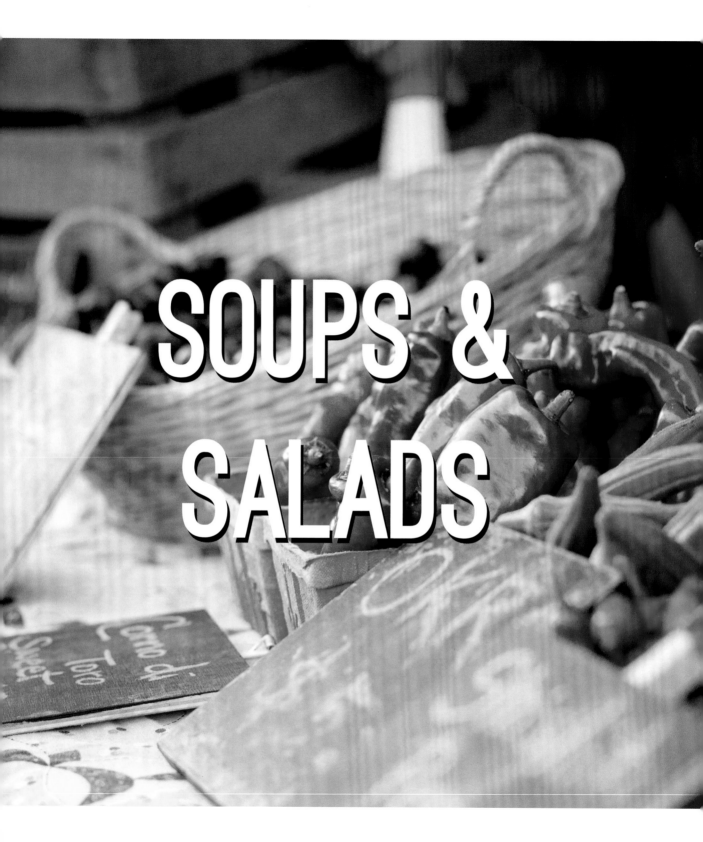

SOUPS & SALADS

fresh & wholesome

Just because crackers and croutons are taboo, doesn't mean saying goodbye to the comfort of hot soup. Soups have become a great monotony-breaker and are so versatile. Use for lunches, as a quick dinner, and a take along food. A thermal-insulated stainless steel mug will allow you to heat soup at home and keep it hot for several hours. This is an excellent option if you are out and about with slim hopes of finding special foods.

Beautiful, colorful salads! I've been a huge fan of salads for most of my life, because of the variety of combinations, the fresh vegetables, and the array of flavorful dressings and add-ins. My vegetable garden becomes my best friend in the springtime as tender lettuce and new spinach curls into growth. Late summer produces the king of the garden—red orbs of sun-ripened tomatoes. If you don't have a garden, consider a small raised bed for a salad and herb garden, or shop farmer's markets through the summer months for locally grown vegetables. The quality and flavor is really just so much better that it will give you a whole new take on the salad bowl! I have included only my basic favorites in this section, but you can create a big variety of salads within the low glycemic diet. Watch out for non-veggie add-ins, and learn to know your dressing options. Ranch dressing is always in style for my girl, but I prefer homemade versions, which are a cinch to make in a blender.

RANCH CHICKEN FAJITA SALAD

This is a great main dish salad on those summer evenings when it's too hot to cook.

2 cups cooked chicken, cubed
½ teaspoon Fajita Seasoning (see Index)
½ teaspoon Taco Seasoning (see Index)
½ cup kidney or black beans
1 small tomato, chopped
¼ cup ranch dressing
2 cups lettuce
¾ cup shredded cheddar cheese

Combine all ingredients except lettuce and cheese; refrigerate.

When ready to serve, divide lettuce on 2 individual serving salad plates. Divide chicken mixture between the 2 plates and top with shredded cheese.

Makes 2 Servings

NUTRITIONAL FACTS

Serving Size 2 Cups

Amount per serving:

Calories 618

Total Fat 35.1g

Total Carbohydrate 15.7g

Dietary Fiber 6g

Sugars 5g

Protein 58.9g

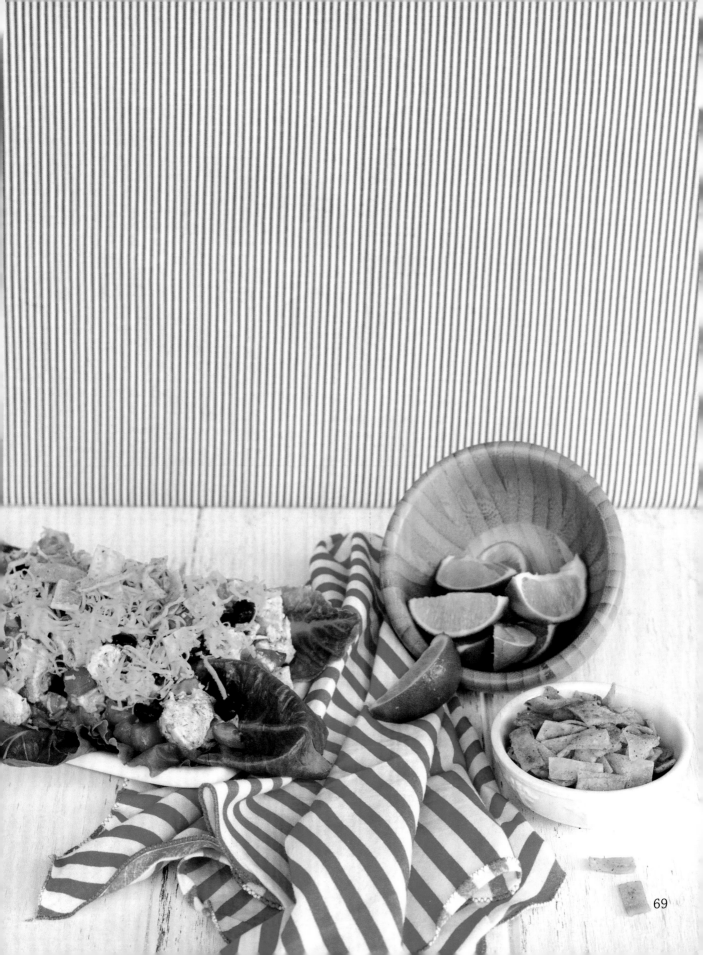

69

QUESADILLA SALAD

This recipe uses leftover cheese quesadillas as a unique and delicious main dish salad. You might end up making a few extra quesadillas just for this purpose!

1 cup lettuce or spinach
¼ cup shredded cheddar cheese
2 tablespoons shredded carrots
2 tablespoons bell pepper or sweet banana pepper, chopped
1 small tomato, chopped
½ Cheese Quesadilla (see Index under variation of Chicken Quesadilla), broken into small pieces
2 tablespoons ranch dressing

On individual serving plate, layer ingredients in order given. Top with dressing and enjoy!

Makes 1 Serving

NUTRITIONAL FACTS

Serving Size 1 Salad

Amount per serving:

Calories 470

Total Fat 31.4g

Total Carbohydrate 24.9g

Dietary Fiber 12g

Sugars 6g

Protein 20.5g

TACO SALAD

1 pound ground beef, fried
8 ounces Refried Beans (see Index)
4 tablespoons Taco Seasoning (see Index)
1 cup Cheese Sauce (see Index)
Shredded lettuce
Chopped tomatoes
4 tablespoons sour cream for serving, optional

Combine beef, beans, and taco seasoning. Heat thoroughly.

Spoon onto 4 individual plates, and top each with 1/4 cup warmed cheese sauce. Serve with chopped vegetables and sour cream, if desired.

Makes 4 Servings

TIPS TO TRY

Andria especially loved this with 2 or 3 crushed chips on top. I used Beanitos® or baked lentil chips.

NUTRITIONAL FACTS

Serving Size 2 Cups

Amount per serving:

Calories 374

Total Fat 23.6g

Total Carbohydrate 13.4g

Dietary Fiber 4g

Sugars 3g

Protein 27.1g

71

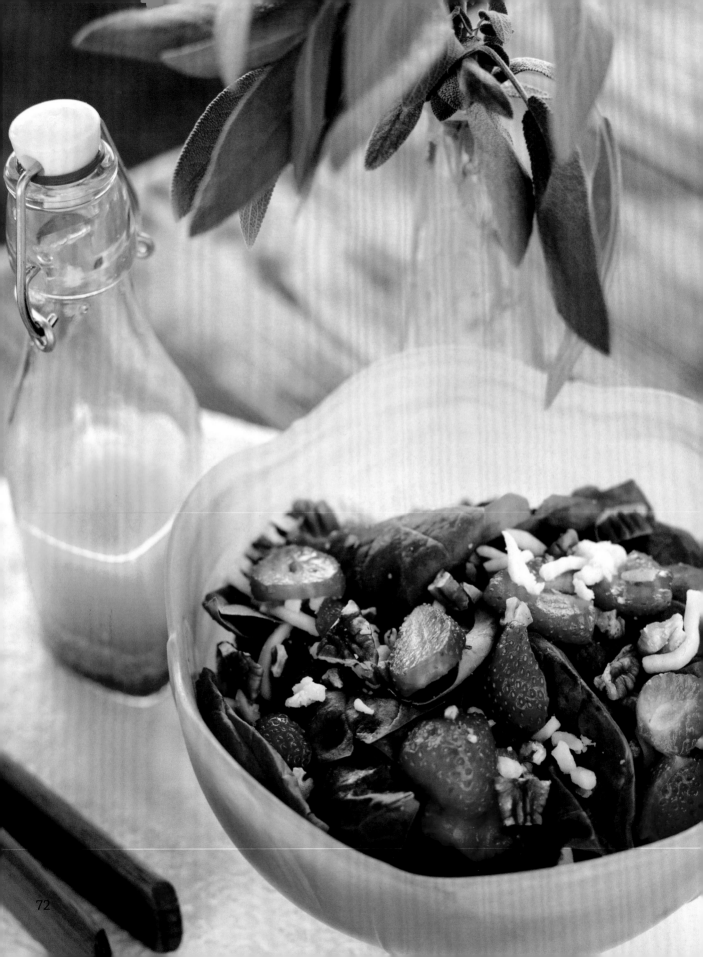

STRAWBERRY SPINACH SALAD

This lovely salad is a spring-time favorite.

Dressing ingredients:
2 tablespoons sesame seeds
¼ teaspoon paprika
¼ teaspoon Worcestershire sauce
12 drops liquid sucralose
½ cup olive oil
¼ cup vinegar
1 teaspoon sea salt

Salad:
2 cups fresh strawberries, sliced
1 (6 oz.) bag baby spinach
¾ cup shredded mozzarella cheese
¼ cup chopped pecans, toasted

Blend dressing ingredients with immersion blender or blender; chill slightly.

Tear spinach into medium sized pieces and toss with remaining salad ingredients. Just before serving, drizzle dressing over salad and mix gently.

Makes 8 Servings

NUTRITIONAL FACTS

Serving Size 1 Cup	
Amount per serving:	
Calories 205	
Total Fat 19.4g	
Total Carbohydrate 5.2g	
Dietary Fiber 2g	
Sugars 2g	
Protein 3.9g	

ANGEL FRUIT SALAD

Fast, easy, light and cool! A perfect summer salad or dessert when fresh fruit is in season.

8 ounces cottage cheese
1½ teaspoons sugar free raspberry gelatin
1 cup Real Whipped Cream (see Index)
1½ cups fresh, mixed berries—blueberries and chopped strawberries

In medium sized bowl, stir cottage cheese and gelatin until well mixed. Add Real Whipped Cream and stir gently.

Just before serving, add fresh, cold berries. Stir to combine. Serve immediately.

Makes 5 Servings

NUTRITIONAL FACTS

Serving Size 1/2 Cup

Amount per serving:

Calories 175

Total Fat 13.7g

Total Carbohydrate 8.1g

Dietary Fiber 1g

Sugars 5g

Protein 6.1g

FINGER JELL-O®

A tried and true snack for children, this became a lunch box staple and is an all around great finger food.

1 tablespoon or 1 package unflavored gelatin
⅓ cup cold water
1 (0.3 oz.) box sugar free gelatin, any flavor
1⅓ cups boiling water

In small bowl, combine unflavored gelatin and cold water.

In second medium sized bowl, mix flavored gelatin and boiling water. Add unflavored gelatin mixture immediately and stir until well dissolved.

Pour into small, shallow square pan and refrigerate until firm. Cut into 2" squares.

Makes 4 Servings

TIPS TO TRY

Finger Jell-O® can also be served as a snack in individual cups. For this, make 2 or more flavors of gelatin. When set, cut into 1" cubes, and mix the cubes into a rainbow of colors in serving cups. Garnish with a party toothpick for serving.

NUTRITIONAL FACTS

Serving Size 1/2 Cup

Amount per serving:

Calories 14

Total Fat 0g

Total Carbohydrate 0.8g

Dietary Fiber 0g

Sugars 0g

Protein 2.8g

RAINBOW JELL-O® BLOCKS

A party must have, rainbow Jell-O® adds a punch of color to any theme or décor. Although this is a simple process, the chilling and layering take time and patience, so plan ahead.

1 (0.3 oz.) box sugar free strawberry gelatin
1 (0.3 oz.) box sugar free lime gelatin
1 (0.3 oz.) box sugar free orange gelatin
1 (0.3 oz.) box sugar free lemon gelatin
2 cups boiling water, divided
2 cups cold water, divided
1 cup sour cream, divided

Mix strawberry gelatin with 1/2 cup boiling water. Stir until dissolved. Add 1/2 cup cold water. Pour 2/3 cup gelatin mixture into 9" glass square pan, reserving remaining strawberry gelatin for next step. Chill until set.

Meanwhile, stir 1/4 cup sour cream into reserved strawberry gelatin, whisking until smooth and totally combined. When first layer is set, gently pour sour cream gelatin on top. Refrigerate.

Using same ratio of water and gelatin, mix lime gelatin. Allow to cool for 20 minutes to avoid melting bottom layer of gelatin, before layering on top of sour cream mixture.

Repeat, chilling and mixing orange and lemon flavors.

When finished, you will have 8 different shades of layered gelatin. When completely firm, cut into squares.

Makes 16 Servings

TIPS TO TRY

This gelatin is easy to turn into a seasonal food, using color themes for holidays.

NUTRITIONAL FACTS

Serving Size 1/3 Cup	
Amount per serving:	
Calories 31	
Total Fat 2.4g	
Total Carbohydrate 1.1g	
Dietary Fiber 0g	
Sugars 0g	
Protein 1.5g	

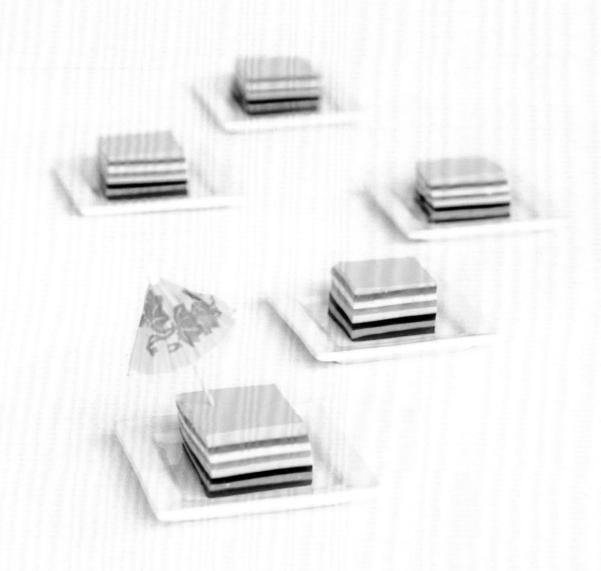

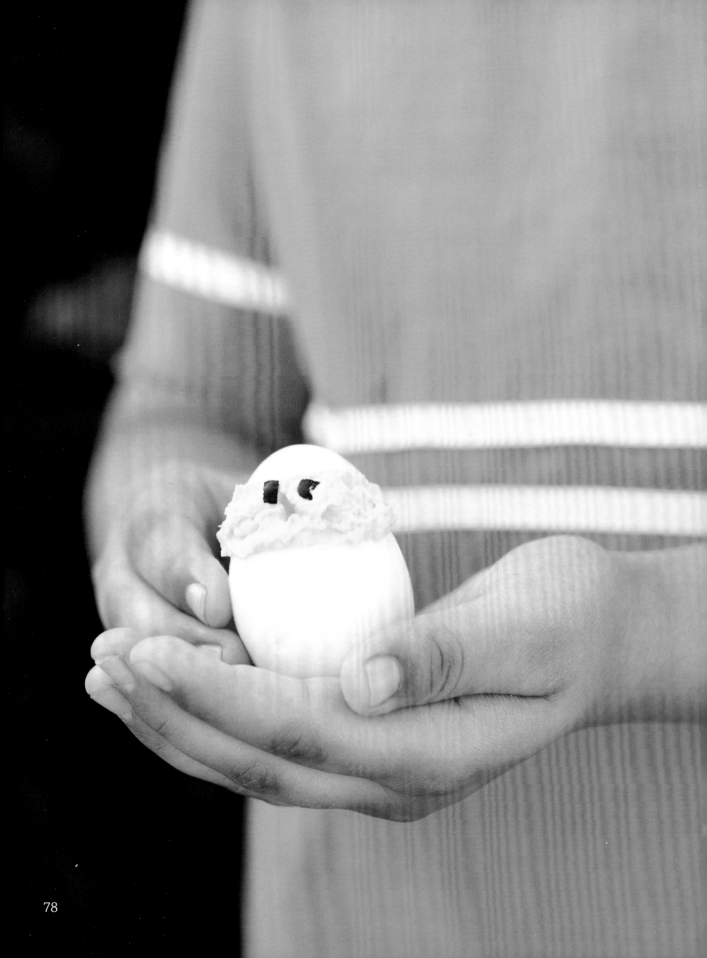

DEVILED EGGS

2 hard boiled eggs, cooled and peeled
2 tablespoons salad dressing
2 tablespoons sour cream
½ teaspoon prepared mustard
¼ teaspoon sea salt
¼ teaspoon freshly ground pepper

Slice eggs in half lengthwise. Remove yolks and place in small bowl. Smash yolks with fork until fine and crumbly. Add salad dressing, sour cream, mustard, salt and pepper. Mix again with fork.

With spoon, divide filling among the 4 halves of eggs. Sprinkle with paprika for garnish.

Makes 2 Servings

Variation: Ranch Bacon Deviled Eggs
Substitute 2 tablespoons ranch dressing for salad dressing and add 1 tablespoon fried bacon, crumbled. Prepare as directed.

TIPS TO TRY

To create chick as pictured, cut 1/4 of egg off the top of hard boiled egg and set aside. With small spoon, scoop yolk section out of white and follow directions for mixing filling. Spoon into hollowed part of egg. Replace top of egg. Garnish chick using pieces of black olive for eyes and shredded carrot for nose.

NUTRITIONAL FACTS

Serving Size 2 Halves	
Amount per serving:	
Calories 136	
Total Fat 11.2g	
Total Carbohydrate 2.8g	
Dietary Fiber 1g	
Sugars 2g	
Protein 6.6g	

CRISPY TORTILLA STRIPS

Tortilla strips are great as a substitute for crackers in any kind of soup. Make a large portion and keep in the freezer for emergency soup days.

1 low carb 8" tortilla
1 tablespoon butter
¼ teaspoon Fajita Seasoning (see Index)

With kitchen shears or sharp knife, cut tortilla in half, then each half into 1/4" strips.

Melt butter in skillet and add tortilla strips. Sprinkle with Fajita Seasoning. Fry over low heat for 5–8 minutes, stirring once every minute to keep from scorching. When strips begin to brown, remove from heat and cool.

Makes 2 Servings

Crispy Tortilla Strips pictured on pg. 69.

NUTRITIONAL FACTS

Serving Size 1/2 Tortilla

Amount per serving:

Calories 96

Total Fat 5.8g

Total Carbohydrate 7g

Dietary Fiber 5g

Sugars 0g

Protein 2.6g

VEGETABLE SOUP

I have been making this soup for several years and knew I had hit a gold mine with a vegetable soup that my little ones actually ate. The secret is that some of the vegetables are pulsed in the blender and hidden from picky eaters. Although the original recipe included potatoes and alphabet pasta, when I substitute with barley and refried beans, the soup is just as delicious.

½ cup carrots, finely chopped
¼ cup pearled barley
1 cup Refried Beans (see Index)
1½ quarts tomato juice, divided
2 celery ribs, chopped
1 small onion, chopped
1½ cups water, divided
Pinch of powdered stevia
1 tablespoon sea salt
1 tablespoon paprika
½ pound ground beef, fried

Combine carrots and pearled barley in saucepan. Add 1 cup water and bring to boil. Simmer on low heat until barley is puffed and tender; about 20 minutes. Remove from heat and drain water.

Meanwhile, cut celery and onion into large chunks and place in another saucepan with 1/2 cup water. Bring to boil, then reduce heat and simmer until soft.

Remove from heat and drain. Place in blender with 2 cups tomato juice. Blend on high speed until celery and onion are smooth.

In large saucepan, combine veggies, barley, remaining tomato juice, and all other ingredients. Heat to boiling, then simmer until ready to serve.

Makes 8 Servings

NUTRITIONAL FACTS

Serving Size 1 Cup

Amount per serving:

Calories 139

Total Fat 4.8g

Total Carbohydrate 16.9g

Dietary Fiber 3g

Sugars 8g

Protein 8.8g

CHICKEN BACON CHOWDER

A mainstay in the line of soups. The cheese sauce thickens the soup and gives it a creamy texture.

¼ cup carrots, diced
¾ cup chicken broth
½ cup Cheese Sauce (see Index)
1 cup cooked chicken, cubed
¼ cup heavy whipping cream
Sea salt and freshly ground pepper, to taste
¼ cup fried bacon, crumbled

In small saucepan, cook carrots in chicken broth until tender. Add all remaining ingredients and bring to gentle simmer. Serve hot.

Makes 3 Servings

NUTRITIONAL FACTS

Serving Size 1 Cup	
Amount per serving:	
Calories 316	
Total Fat 22.8g	
Total Carbohydrate 4.5g	
Dietary Fiber 0g	
Sugars 3g	
Protein 22.9g	

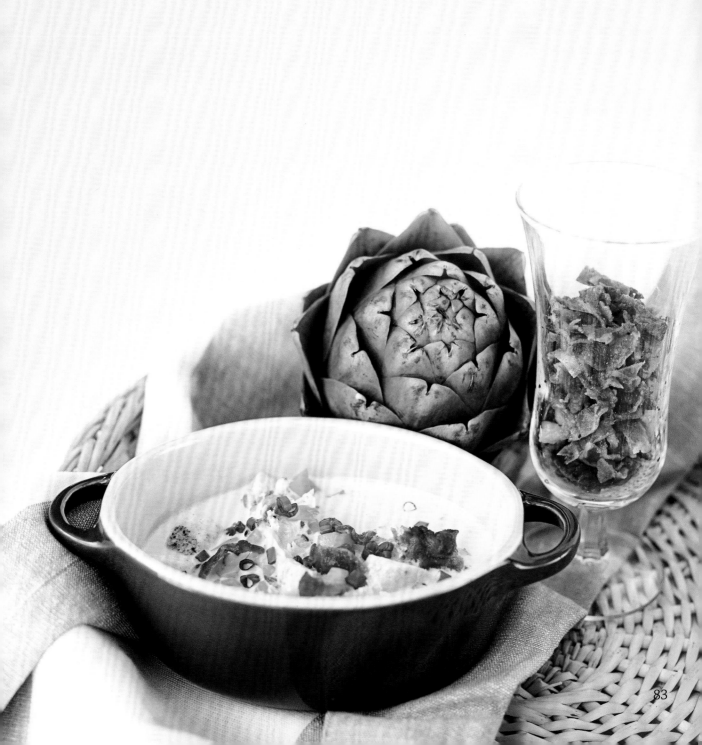

CHICKEN BARLEY SOUP

Made in a slow cooker or on the stove top, this is the ultimate in chicken soup comfort food.

1½ cups water, divided
¾ cup minced carrots
½ cup minced celery
¼ cup minced onion
¼ cup pearled barley
1 pound cooked chicken, cubed
2 cups chicken broth
1 bay leaf
¼ teaspoon cumin
½ teaspoon sea salt
½ teaspoon freshly ground pepper

In large saucepan, combine 1 cup water, carrots, celery, onion, and barley. Bring to a boil, then simmer until veggies and barley are tender, approximately 20 minutes.

Add remaining 1/2 cup water and all additional ingredients. Simmer for 20–30 minutes.

Remove and discard bay leaf. Serve with Crispy Tortilla Strips (see Index), if desired.

Makes 5 Servings

TIPS TO TRY

To make soup in slow cooker: simmer veggies and barley only 10 minutes. Pour into slow cooker and add remaining ingredients. Heat on low for 5 hours.

NUTRITIONAL FACTS

Serving Size 1 Cup
Amount per serving:
Calories 168
Total Fat 7.4g
Total Carbohydrate 7g
Dietary Fiber 1g
Sugars 1g
Protein 26.2g

CABBAGE BEEF SOUP

1 rib celery, finely chopped
1 onion, finely chopped
1 pound ground beef
½ teaspoon garlic powder
¼ teaspoon freshly ground pepper
1 (15 oz.) can red or black beans
¼ head cabbage, finely shredded
1 quart chicken broth
1 teaspoon Taco Seasoning (see Index)

In large kettle, brown beef with onions and celery until veggies are tender. Drain. Add all other ingredients and simmer on low heat for 1 hour.

Serve with sour cream.

Makes 8 Servings

NUTRITIONAL FACTS

Serving Size 1 Cup

Amount per serving:

Calories 192

Total Fat 9.2g

Total Carbohydrate 12.7g

Dietary Fiber 4g

Sugars 3g

Protein 14.6g

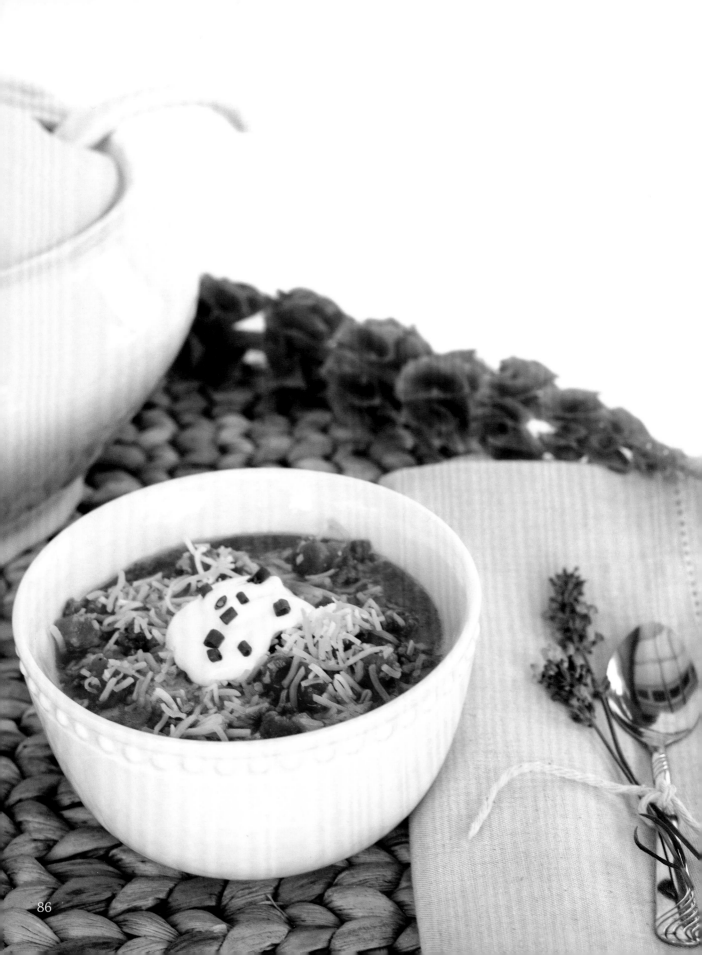

SOUPER DUPER CHILI

Hearty and spicy, you really can't go wrong with chili. Adjust the chili powder and cayenne pepper to the heat you prefer. The best thing about chili is that it can be made in large amounts, then frozen in portions for future use.

1 pound sausage or ground beef, fried
1 (15 oz.) can chunk tomatoes
8 ounces salsa
1 (15 oz.) can kidney or pinto beans
1 pint tomato juice
¾ teaspoon chili powder
½ teaspoon freshly ground pepper
½ teaspoon sea salt
¼ teaspoon cayenne pepper, optional
Sour cream and shredded cheddar cheese, optional

Pour all ingredients (except sour cream and cheese) into large kettle. Heat until mixture is boiling, then reduce heat and simmer for 30 minutes.

Slow Cooker Method: Pour all ingredients into 4 quart slow cooker. Heat on low for 4 hours.

Serve with sour cream and shredded cheddar cheese, or Crispy Tortilla Strips (see Index).

Makes 7 Servings

NUTRITIONAL FACTS

Serving Size 1 Cup	
Amount per serving:	
Calories 318	
Total Fat 20.9g	
Total Carbohydrate 19.5g	
Dietary Fiber 5g	
Sugars 8g	
Protein 14.6g	

CONDENSED MUSHROOM SOUP

I was thrilled to discover this cream soup with no milk ingredients. I use it sparingly or thin it with water or cream to stretch the carb limits on the beans, but it works great as a sauce for any main dish, especially when used with cheese.

1 onion, chopped
1 tablespoon olive oil
2 tablespoons fresh herbs, chopped, or 2 teaspoon dried,
crushed herbs of choice (sage, thyme, rosemary, or parsley)
½ teaspoon freshly ground pepper
4 cups fresh mushrooms, sliced
1 (15 oz.) can white kidney beans, drained
1 tablespoon soy sauce
2 tablespoons nutritional yeast (optional)

Sauté chopped onion in olive oil. Add herbs and pepper; sauté until onion is clear. Add mushrooms and cook 4 minutes.

Purée in blender with beans until smooth. Add soy sauce and blend well.

Makes 4 Servings

TIPS TO TRY

Make a batch of this soup and freeze in small portions for use in cooking.

NUTRITIONAL FACTS

Serving Size 1/2 Cup	
Amount per serving:	
Calories 144	
Total Fat 3.7g	
Total Carbohydrate 20.5g	
Dietary Fiber 6g	
Sugars 4g	
Protein 9.3g	

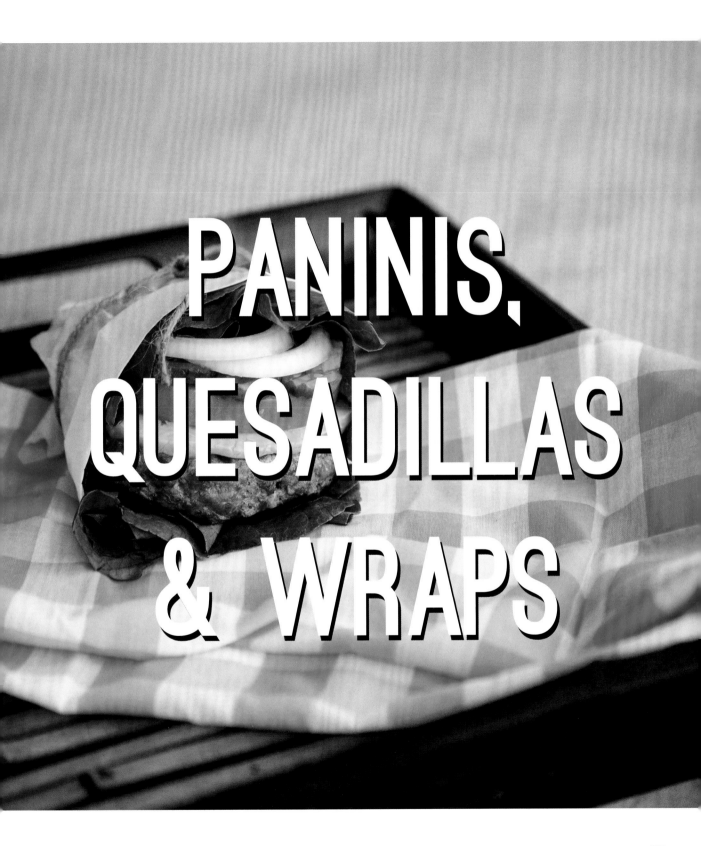

PANINIS, QUESADILLAS & WRAPS

that's a wrap

The day I discovered the low carbohydrate tortilla, the entire low glycemic index world opened up! Tortillas are an excellent option because they are like a piece of bread, just much, much thinner, which equals fewer carbs. Because they pair well with sour cream and shredded cheese, no one misses the rich gravies and sauces. I cannot cook without a pack of tortillas in the pantry and two more in the freezer for back up! They freeze very well.

My recipes are geared toward child friendly wrap combinations, but feel free to concoct your own favorite food combinations. Wraps are a great way to use leftovers that really are not enough for a meal in themselves.

Although paninis are relatively new on the food scene, there is a good reason for their popularity. I found the method of fixing paninis especially appealing when making the drastic switch from sandwiches with home made white bread to low carb flatbread (much less texture and flat, bland taste). Heating or grilling the flatbread with a spritz of olive oil does wonders! When cooking chicken or beef for entrées, make extra for fillings for these unbeatable sandwiches.

HOT DOG TOSTADOS

What isn't to love in this childhood favorite? The bonus is that with the tortilla and cheese, no one will miss the bun.

2 low carb 8" tortillas
2 hot dogs, cut into ½" slices
4 tablespoons Sugar Free Pizza Sauce or 3 tablespoons
Homemade Ketchup (see Index)
¼ cup shredded mozzarella cheese

Preheat oven to 350°. Place tortillas flat on baking sheet. Top each tortilla with 1 sliced hot dog, 2 tablespoons Sugar Free Pizza Sauce, and a sprinkle of cheese.

Bake for 10-12 minutes or until tortillas are crisp and cheese is melted. Cut into wedges to serve.

Makes 2 Servings

TIPS TO TRY

This is a great after school snack. To quick prep: slice hot dog and heat in microwave. Preheat broiler to high. Spread tortilla with pizza sauce, hot dog, and cheese. Place under broiler for 3 minutes or until cheese melts.

NUTRITIONAL FACTS

Serving Size 1 Tostada	
Amount per serving:	
Calories	356
Total Fat	22.3g
Total Carbohydrate	16.8g
Dietary Fiber	9g
Sugars	2g
Protein	18.3g

OVEN CHICKEN QUESADILLAS

A teen style meal! Pop chicken quesadillas into the oven anytime you have leftover chicken in the refrigerator for a tasty, light supper or a quick pick me up.

2½ cups cooked chicken, cubed
⅔ cup salsa
¾ teaspoon cumin
½ teaspoon oregano
6 low carb 8" tortillas
¾ cup shredded mozzarella cheese
6 tablespoons Sugar Free Pizza Sauce (see Index)
Chopped onions and peppers, optional
1 tablespoon butter, softened

Preheat oven to 450°. Combine chicken, salsa, cumin, and oregano.

Stir gently. Butter 1 side of each tortilla. With buttered side up, place 3 tortillas on a greased baking sheet. Spread approximately 3/4 cup chicken mixture on each one. Place remaining 3 tortillas on top. Spread with pizza sauce, cheese, and veggies if desired.

Bake for 10 minutes. Cut each quesadilla into 6 wedges and serve immediately.

Makes 18 Servings

NUTRITIONAL FACTS

Serving Size 1 Wedge
Amount per serving:
Calories 88
Total Fat 2.6g
Total Carbohydrate 5.8g
Dietary Fiber 4g
Sugars 0g
Protein 9g

CHICKEN QUESADILLAS

Super simple; super speedy! This is one of my husband's standby meals when he's the one doing the cooking.

4 low carb 8" tortillas
1 cup cooked chicken, cubed
1 cup mozzarella or cheddar cheese
Softened butter
Ranch dressing, for dipping

Preheat quesadilla or panini maker. Spread 1 side of each tortilla with butter. With buttered side up, spread with chicken and cheese. Top with second tortilla.

Bake or grill in quesadilla maker until quesadilla is lightly browned and crisp around edges. Remove and cut into 6 wedges. Serve with ranch dressing for dipping.

Makes 4 Servings

TIPS TO TRY

Variation: Cheese Quesadilla: omit the chicken and use only cheese. Serve with salsa.

NUTRITIONAL FACTS

Serving Size 3 Wedges
Amount per serving:
Calories 257
Total Fat 10.4g
Total Carbohydrate 14.6g
Dietary Fiber 9g
Sugars 0g
Protein 22.1g

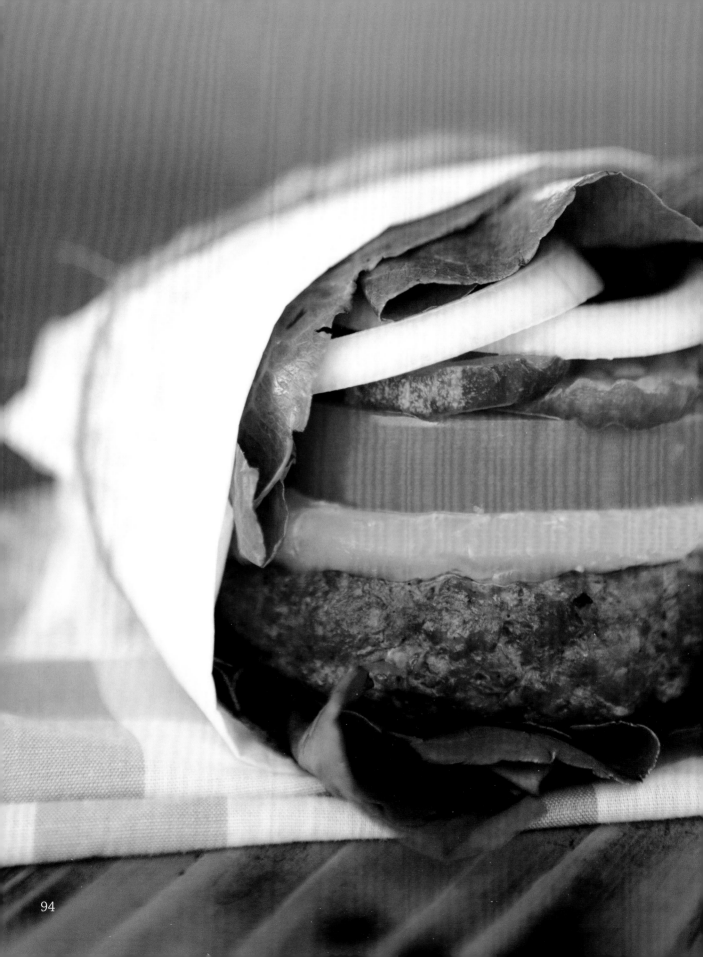

ALL-AMERICAN HAMBURGERS

There's really nothing like that juicy burger, dressed up with all the fixings, or kept simple with a slice of cheese and ketchup. Hamburgers hot off the grill seem to shout summer! The best addition at our house is a thick slice of ripe tomato, fresh from the garden.

1 pound ground beef
1 egg, lightly beaten
½ cup fine bread crumbs (see Index for Almond Meal Dinner Rolls and Bread Crumbs)
2 tablespoons minced onion
½ teaspoon sea salt
½ teaspoon freshly ground pepper

Mix all ingredients in medium sized bowl. With burger press, shape into 6 hamburger patties. Grill over medium heat until burgers reach desired doneness.

Serve with Homemade Ketchup (see Index), mustard, lettuce, and tomato.

Makes 6 Servings

NUTRITIONAL FACTS

Serving Size 1 Patty
Amount per serving:
Calories 243
Total Fat 17.7g
Total Carbohydrate 3.5g
Dietary Fiber 2g
Sugars 1g
Protein 17.6g

PERFECT PANINIS

Paninis were a real hit when I stumbled onto the discovery of using a low carb flatbread. I use a George Foreman® indoor grill in place of a panini maker with excellent results.

For each of the following recipes, you will need:
4 slices of flatbread

Mushroom Cheese Panini:
1 pound ground beef, fried
¼ cup chopped onion, optional
2 ounces cream cheese
½ cup Condensed Mushroom Soup (see Index)
Sliced cheddar cheese

Pizza Burger Panini:
1 pound ground beef, fried
Sautéed onions and peppers, optional
1 cup Sugar Free Pizza Sauce (see Index)
12 slices pepperoni
Shredded mozzarella cheese

Chicken Bacon Panini:
1½ cups cooked chicken, cubed
2 tablespoons cream cheese
1 tablespoon ranch dressing
¼ cup fried bacon, crumbled
Shredded mozzarella cheese

Fill one half of each flatbread with meat filling, add cheese, and top with other half of flatbread.

Preheat indoor grill or panini maker. Before cooking on grill, spritz top of sandwich with olive oil. Cook approximately 5 minutes or until heated through.

Makes 4 Servings (per recipe)

Nutritional Facts for the Pizza Burger Panini and the Chicken Bacon Panini can be found on page 187.

TIPS TO TRY

Make a large batch of paninis at once. When cooled, wrap individually and freeze for a quick meal later. Simply pop in microwave and reheat.

NUTRITIONAL FACTS *

Serving Size 1 Panini (Mush.)
Amount per serving:
Calories 535
Total Fat 35.1g
Total Carbohydrate 22g
Dietary Fiber 9g
Sugars 2g
Protein 38.3g

CHICKEN SALAD TORTILLA WRAPS

These wraps have become a picnic staple for our family. Add chilies or jalapeños for a zesty punch.

¼ cup salad dressing
¼ cup sour cream
1 hard boiled egg, chopped
1 teaspoon prepared mustard
Sea salt and freshly ground pepper, to taste
2 cups cooked chicken, cubed
¼ cup shredded cheddar cheese
4 low carb 8" tortillas
2 tablespoons fried bacon, crumbled, optional
Lettuce and tomato, optional

In small bowl, combine salad dressing, sour cream, egg, mustard, salt, and pepper. Add chicken and cheese; stir gently to combine.

Divide evenly among 4 tortillas. Add bacon, lettuce, and tomato just before serving; sprinkle with additional salt and pepper. Fold and wrap tortilla.

Makes 4 Servings

NUTRITIONAL FACTS

Serving Size 1 Wrap

Amount per serving:

Calories 338

Total Fat 14.2g

Total Carbohydrate 16.7g

Dietary Fiber 9g

Sugars 1g

Protein 31.7g

COLD CUT WRAPS

Great lunch box or picnic fare, cold cut wraps go anywhere with your choice of filling.

2 low carb 8" tortillas
8 slices deli ham
4 slices cheddar cheese
Sea salt and freshly ground pepper, to taste
Shredded lettuce, chopped tomatoes, and bacon, optional

Dressing:
1 tablespoon mayonnaise
2 tablespoons sour cream
½ teaspoon Taco Seasoning (see Index)

Mix dressing ingredients in small bowl with spoon. Spread over tortillas.

Top each tortilla with 4 slices ham and 2 slices cheese. Sprinkle with salt and pepper. Add lettuce, tomato, and bacon, if desired.

Fold and wrap tortilla.

Makes 2 Servings

NUTRITIONAL FACTS

Serving Size 1 Wrap

Amount per serving:

Calories 543

Total Fat 32.6g

Total Carbohydrate 20.4g

Dietary Fiber 11g

Sugars 1g

Protein 37.8g

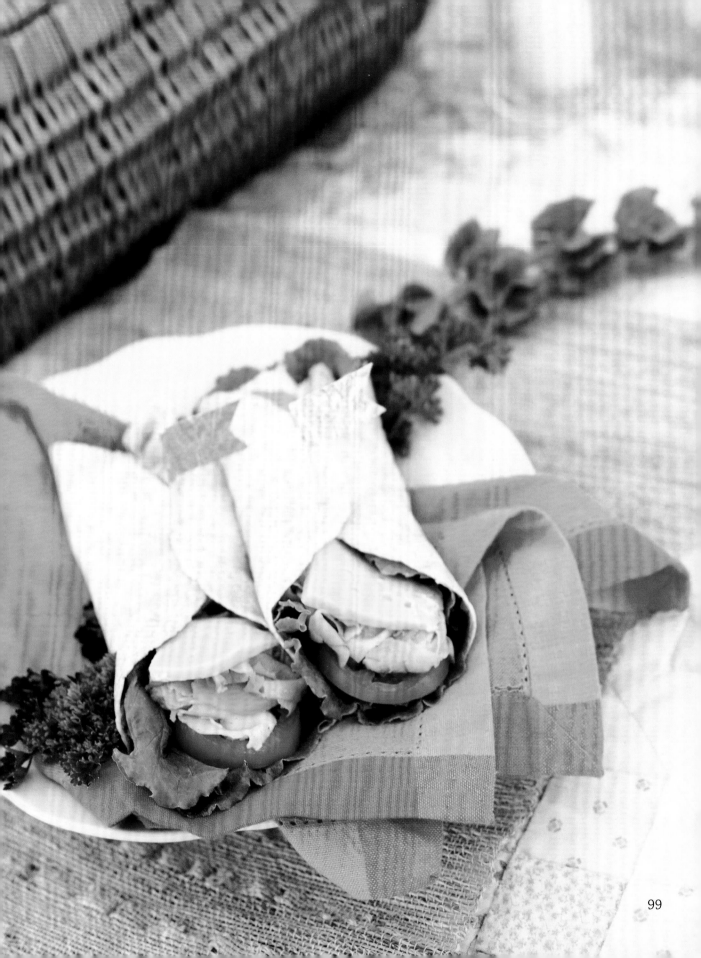

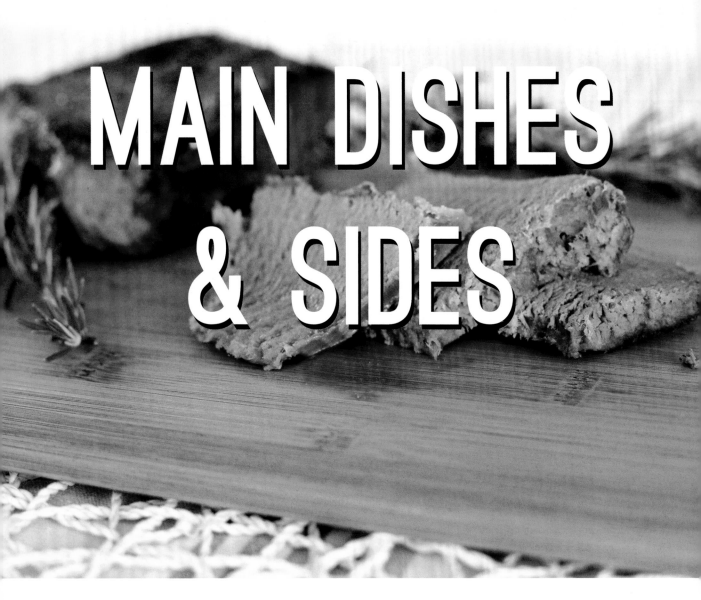

MAIN DISHES & SIDES

the main event

Here it is—the crux of your cooking! Because of the tremendous need for protein, this part of every meal is essential. Without it, one hour after mealtime your child may be begging for food, and you will deal with what I term "snack stress". The good news is that, equipped with knowledge and planning, mealtimes will become a main event again, not five minutes of grabbing something light and fast.

The big thing, and I mean the *really big thing* here, is meat. You will want to buy in bulk if you are not doing so already. I have found chicken to be the most versatile. Chicken legs, thighs, breasts, boneless, bone-in, whole roasting hens... you get the picture.

The slow cooker is an excellent tool in cutting down on actual hands-on cooking time. Again, the key to ease is planning ahead. I found it much easier to cook dinner when the meat was thawed in the refrigerator and ready to go. Learning to cook with garlic and herbs (dried or fresh) opens a new world of flavor in main dishes. With so much from one food group, variety becomes your secret weapon against mealtime doldrums.

BAKED CHICKEN NUGGETS

A fun twist on the classic favorite. I also do nuggets on my George Foreman® indoor grill for a change of pace from the oven version.

½ **cup grated parmesan cheese**
½ **teaspoon Seasoned Salt (see Index)**
¼ **teaspoon freshly ground pepper**
½ **teaspoon Fajita Seasoning (see Index)**
4 **boneless, skinless chicken breasts, cut into nugget sized pieces**
½ **cup melted butter**

Preheat oven to 400°. Line baking sheet with foil, then spray liberally with nonstick cooking spray.

Combine dry ingredients in shallow bowl. Dip chicken in melted butter and then sprinkle with seasoning mixture.

Place on baking sheet. Bake for 20-25 minutes or until nuggets are golden. Serve with ranch dressing for dipping.

Makes 4 Servings

TIPS TO TRY

Chicken will cut easily when still half frozen.

NUTRITIONAL FACTS

Serving Size 4 Ounces

Amount per serving:

Calories 380

Total Fat 28.9g

Total Carbohydrate 0.4g

Dietary Fiber 0g

Sugars 0g

Protein 29.1g

GRILLED DIJON CHICKEN

1-2 tablespoons olive oil
¾ cup low carb vanilla yogurt
2 tablespoons Dijon mustard
2 tablespoons chopped fresh dill
Sea salt and freshly ground pepper, to taste, divided
1 pound boneless, skinless chicken thighs

Preheat outdoor grill and lightly brush rack with oil.

In small bowl mix yogurt, mustard, dill, salt, and pepper. Set aside.

Rinse chicken with cold water and pat dry with paper towels. Place on a plate and brush all sides with oil. Sprinkle with salt and pepper.

Grill chicken approximately 12 minutes on each side, or until meat thermometer inserted in thickest part of meat reads 165° and juices run clear.

Serve with mustard sauce.

Makes 4 Servings

NUTRITIONAL FACTS

Serving Size 4 Ounces

Amount per serving:

Calories 187

Total Fat 8.8g

Total Carbohydrate 1.4g

Dietary Fiber 0g

Sugars 1g

Protein 24.2g

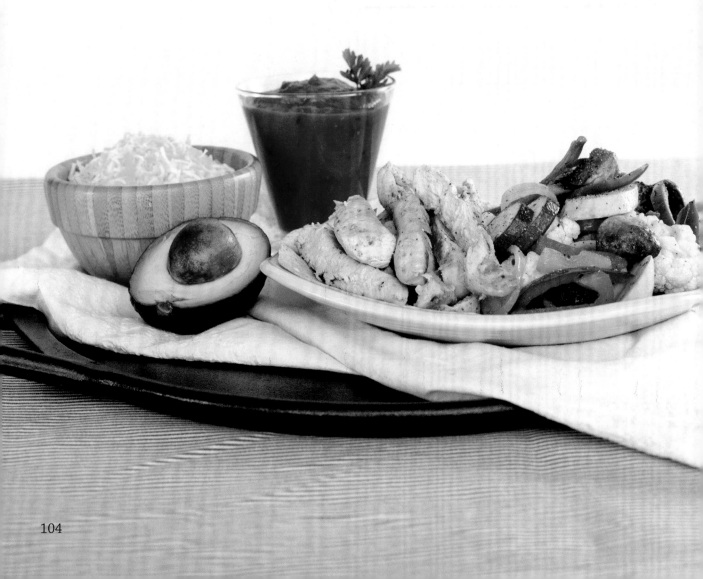

CHICKEN FAJITAS

3 tablespoons olive oil, divided
2 tablespoons lemon juice
2 tablespoons Fajita Seasoning (see Index)
1½ pounds boneless, skinless chicken breast, cut into strips
½ red pepper, diced or cut into strips
½ green pepper, diced or cut into strips
½ onion, diced or cut into strips
Sour cream and shredded cheese, optional

Combine 2 tablespoons olive oil, lemon juice and Fajita Seasoning and pour over chicken breast. Marinate in refrigerator 4 hours or overnight.

In large skillet, sauté vegetables in remaining 1 tablespoon olive oil until medium tender. Remove from skillet and keep warm. In same skillet, fry chicken over medium heat until juices run clear.

Return veggies to skillet; heat through. Serve on warmed, low carb 8" tortillas with sour cream and shredded cheese if desired.

Makes 8 Servings

Nutritional analysis does not include the low carb tortilla, sour cream, or cheese. Be sure to add in carb amounts for optional ingredients.

TIPS TO TRY

Vegetable Stir Fry (see Index) makes an excellent side with this meal.

NUTRITIONAL FACTS *

Serving Size 1/2 Cup
Amount per serving:
Calories 241
Total Fat 9.1g
Total Carbohydrate 1.7g
Dietary Fiber 0g
Sugars 1g
Protein 25.5g

FAJITA MARINADE FOR CHICKEN OR STEAK

This is my most used marinade recipe. Our family loves this combination of herbs and flavors.

½ cup olive oil
½ cup white vinegar
2 teaspoons oregano
2 teaspoons chili powder
1 clove garlic
½ teaspoon sea salt
½ teaspoon freshly ground pepper
½ onion, thinly sliced, optional
1 red or green pepper, thinly sliced, optional
1½ pounds chicken breast or steak

In blender or food processer, combine oil, vinegar, oregano, chili powder, garlic, salt, and pepper. Pour into large skillet; sauté onion and peppers with marinade mixture until veggies are semi-soft. Cool.

Place whole pieces of meat in shallow baking pan and cover with marinade/veggie mixture. Marinate in refrigerator 6 hours or overnight.

Remove meat from marinade. For steak: grill to desired done-ness. For chicken breast: grill until meat thermometer inserted into thickest part of chicken reads 165° and juices run clear. With chef's knife, slice meat into thin strips before serving.

To stir fry: Cut raw meat into thin strips. Place in shallow baking pan and cover with marinade/veggie mixture. Marinate in refrigerator 6 hours or overnight.

Stir fry in large skillet until juices run clear. Serve immediately.

Makes 6 Servings

TIPS TO TRY

If pressed for time, skip the veggies and do only the basic marinade and the meat.

NUTRITIONAL FACTS

Serving Size 4 Ounces

Amount per serving:

Calories 398

Total Fat 24.3g

Total Carbohydrate 0.2g

Dietary Fiber 0g

Sugars 0g

Protein 29.6g

GOURMET CHICKEN

Don't be intimidated by the name of this recipe—it's one of the easiest chicken dishes in my collection of recipes. We love it for Sunday dinner.

½ cup Condensed Mushroom Soup (see Index)
¼ cup heavy whipping cream
2 tablespoons water
¼ cup sour cream
6 boneless, skinless chicken breasts
Sea salt and freshly ground pepper, to taste
6 slices cheddar cheese
1 cup fine bread crumbs (see Index for Almond Meal Dinner Rolls and Bread Crumbs)
¼ cup butter, melted

Preheat oven to 350°. In small bowl, combine mushroom soup, cream, and water. Add sour cream.

In well greased 9x13" baking pan, place chicken breasts in single layer. Sprinkle liberally with salt and pepper. Top each piece with a slice of cheese. Pour mushroom soup/sour cream mixture on top. Sprinkle bread crumbs overall and drizzle with melted butter.

Bake, uncovered, for 1 hour.

Makes 6 Servings

TIPS TO TRY

For an even more gourmet touch, top the chicken with sautéed or canned mushrooms and fried bacon, crumbled.

NUTRITIONAL FACTS

Serving Size 1 Chicken Breast

Amount per serving:

Calories 523

Total Fat 36.1g

Total Carbohydrate 10.5g

Dietary Fiber 4g

Sugars 2g

Protein 38.9g

HERB ROASTED CHICKEN IN BRINE

Ahh…what lovelier aroma than a chicken roasting in the oven? This is one dish I prepare when I am in the house as it bakes, simply to enjoy the delicious smells permeating the kitchen. One tip—plan ahead! I have wanted roasted chicken for dinner only to remember the hen is in the freezer, frozen rock solid. Start 2 days ahead to allow for 1 day of thawing in the refrigerator and 1 day or overnight for soaking. Brined chicken is super juicy, and roasting it at a high temperature produces a delicious, browned skin without drying the meat. On second thought, go ahead and make 2 hens! There's nothing like leftover roasted chicken in the fridge!

Brine:
2 quarts water
½ cup sea salt

1 large roasting hen (approximately 3 pounds)
2 tablespoons olive oil
5 cloves garlic, divided
1 lemon
Sea salt
Freshly ground pepper
Fresh or dried herbs of choice (parsley, basil, oregano, or thyme)

Place thawed chicken in large container. Mix brine and pour over chicken. Refrigerate 3-8 hours or overnight.

Preheat oven to 450°. Place chicken, breast side up, in cast iron skillet or other roasting pan. Rub outside of chicken with olive oil and 3 crushed garlic cloves. Cut lemon in half and place inside cavity of chicken with remaining 2 garlic cloves and herbs of choice. Sprinkle liberally with sea salt and pepper.

Bake for 30 minutes, then reduce oven temperature to 325° and bake for additional 1½ hours, or until meat thermometer reads 165° when inserted in breast of chicken.

Makes 8 Servings

TIPS TO TRY

When using a cast iron skillet, spray with nonstick cooking spray before baking chicken. Cover chicken loosely with foil, then remove foil during last 30 minutes of baking time to allow chicken to brown.

NUTRITIONAL FACTS

Serving Size 3.5 Ounces	
Amount per serving:	
Calories 256	
Total Fat 19.0g	
Total Carbohydrate 1.0g	
Dietary Fiber 0g	
Sugars 0g	
Protein 19.4g	

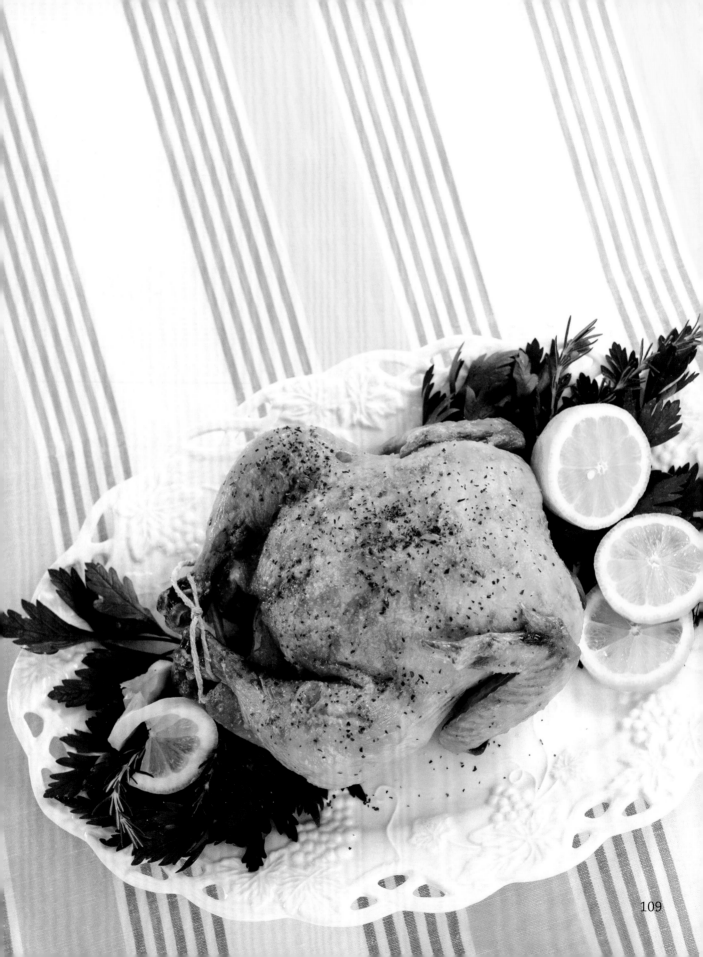

QUICK & EASY SLOW COOKER CHICKEN

Cooking dinner really doesn't get any easier than this tender chicken version. Let the slow cooker do the work while you are out and about.

2 tablespoons olive oil, divided
1 tablespoon lemon juice
1 tablespoon parsley flakes
1 teaspoon celery seed
1 teaspoon Italian seasoning
2 boneless, skinless chicken breasts
1 cup chicken broth

Combine 1 tablespoon olive oil, lemon juice, parsley, celery seed, and Italian seasoning. Pour over chicken and refrigerate 4 hours or overnight.

Remove chicken from marinade and discard marinade. In large skillet, brown chicken lightly in 1 tablespoon olive oil. Place in slow cooker. Pour chicken broth over breasts. Cook on low 4 hours.

Makes 2 Servings

TIPS TO TRY

Serve with lentils and a lettuce salad on the side.

NUTRITIONAL FACTS

Serving Size 1 Chicken Breast

Amount per serving:

Calories 202

Total Fat 10.1g

Total Carbohydrate 1g

Dietary Fiber 0g

Sugars 0g

Protein 25.6g

SUPER CHICKEN & LENTILS

2 boneless, skinless chicken breasts
2 tablespoons olive oil
1 cup lentils or pearled barley
½ cup onions, finely chopped
1 clove garlic, minced
½ teaspoon freshly ground pepper
¾ teaspoon curry powder
¾ teaspoon sea salt
3 cups chicken broth
Sour cream, optional
Mayonnaise, optional

Cut chicken into small pieces and sauté 5 minutes in skillet with oil and lentils or barley. Add onions, garlic, and seasonings, stirring until onions turn clear.

Remove from heat and pour into slow cooker. Add chicken broth. Cook on high for 3 hours or until lentils are soft.

Serve with sour cream or mayonnaise.

Makes 4 Servings

NUTRITIONAL FACTS

Serving Size 1 Cup

Amount per serving:

Calories 260

Total Fat 9.1g

Total Carbohydrate 22.8g

Dietary Fiber 8g

Sugars 3g

Protein 22.4g

111

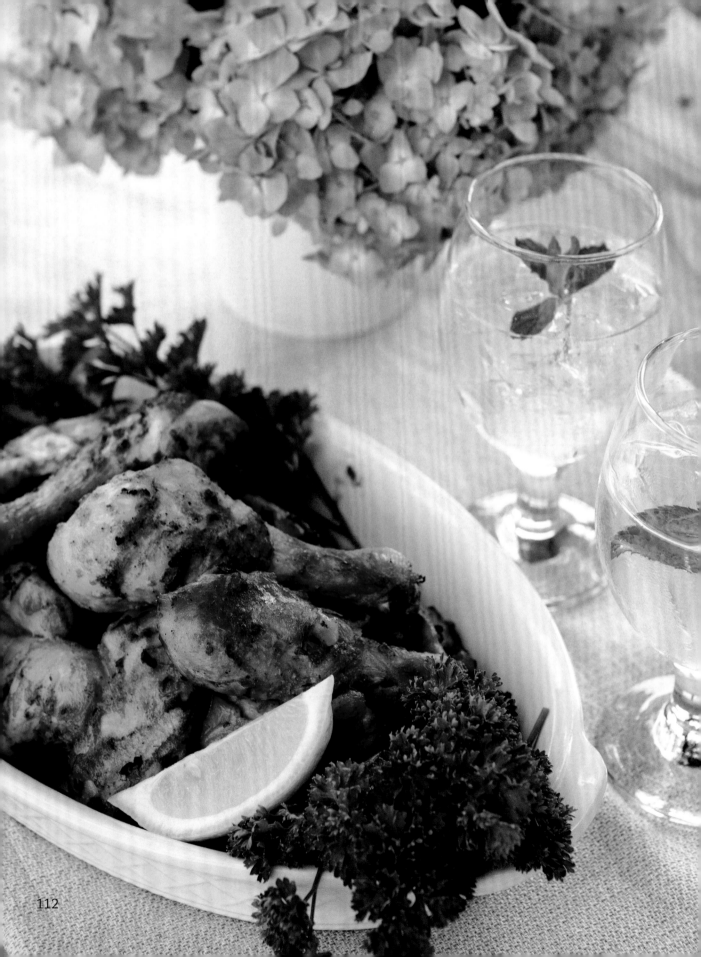

SUMMERTIME BARBECUED CHICKEN

Barbecued chicken on the grill! The sizzling smell takes me back to my growing up years in mid-state New York on a farm. The table was loaded with a full course, summer time spread of fresh veggies from the garden, but the chicken always stole the show! Juicy and succulent, the number of ingredients in the sauce contributes to the delicious combination of flavors incorporated into the meat.

2 cloves garlic
1 small onion
¾ cup celery leaves
1½ cups cold water
½ cup vinegar
1 tablespoon Worcestershire sauce
1½ cups olive oil
2 teaspoons sea salt
¼ teaspoon freshly ground pepper
1 teaspoon celery salt
2 teaspoons Seasoned Salt (see Index)
½ teaspoon oregano
¾ cup Homemade Ketchup (see Index)
1 teaspoon onion salt
¼ teaspoon liquid smoke
5 pounds fresh chicken legs, thighs, or drumsticks

Rinse chicken in cold water; set aside. Place remaining ingredients in blender or food processor and blend until well mixed. Reserve 1 cup sauce. Place chicken in large bowl and pour sauce mixture on top. Refrigerate 6 hours or overnight.

Remove chicken from sauce. Grill chicken over medium heat, basting with reserved sauce, until it reaches desired doneness (165°). Discard used sauce.

Makes 14 Servings

TIPS TO TRY

This is a large recipe and can easily be divided in half. I like to do a large batch of chicken at once, then freeze or refrigerate leftovers for other meals. The possibilities are unlimited. The unused sauce also stores well in the refrigerator.

NUTRITIONAL FACTS

Serving Size 3.5 Ounces	
Amount per serving:	
Calories 473	
Total Fat 38.2g	
Total Carbohydrate 2.5g	
Dietary Fiber 0g	
Sugars 1g	
Protein 28.8g	

MASTER BEAN METHOD

This basic recipe is foolproof, although you need to plan ahead because of the cooking time involved. It couldn't be easier, especially because you can do a large amount at a time and freeze the beans for later use. My favorites are doing chickpeas for homemade hummus and kidney beans for refried beans.

This method works to cook any type of dried beans—kidney beans, black beans, pinto beans, or chickpeas.

Step 1:
Measure 3 cups of beans and rinse thoroughly in cold water.

Step 2:
Place washed and drained beans in large bowl. Cover with 9 cups cold water. Soak overnight.

Step 3:
In the morning, drain the beans. Place in saucepan, cover with water, and bring water to rolling boil. Boil 1 minute. Remove from heat and drain. This step promotes better digestion of the beans.

Step 4:
Place beans in 4–5 quart slow cooker. Cover with cold water. Cook on high for 8–9 hours.

When finished, the beans should be soft when pricked with fork, but not mushy. Drain beans and rinse with cold water until water runs clear.

Makes 24 Servings (6 Cups)

TIPS TO TRY

Cooked beans spoil quickly. Divide beans into meal size portions and freeze until ready to use.

REFRIED BEANS

We love these refried beans. Make a batch and freeze in small portions for use in wraps, soups, and even with eggs and cheese for breakfast. You can reduce or increase the garlic to suit your taste. Beans have a low glycemic index, but are still a significant source of carbohydrate, so watch these serving sizes.

**3 cups cooked beans (use Master Bean Recipe—see Index)
or 2 (15 oz.) cans pinto beans
½ onion, chopped
2 cloves garlic, minced
1 teaspoon cumin
1 teaspoon sea salt
2 tablespoons fresh cilantro, or 2 teaspoons minced, dried cilantro**

In large skillet, mix all ingredients and fry over low heat for 15 minutes, stirring often.

Using immersion blender, blend mixture until nearly smooth. Voilà! Homemade refried beans—not out of the can.

Makes 8 Servings

NUTRITIONAL FACTS

Serving Size 1/4 Cup

Amount per serving:

Calories 84

Total Fat 0.6g

Total Carbohydrate 15.2g

Dietary Fiber 4g

Sugars 1g

Protein 5.0g

SAVORY LENTILS

Any lentils can be used in this recipe, although the light brown ones will tend to use more liquid as they cook versus the red lentils. Try cooking a batch and keeping them in the refrigerator or freezer, then adding to soups, or serving as a side with melted cheese or topped with ranch dressing.

½ onion, chopped
1 garlic clove, minced
½ teaspoon cumin
¾ cup red lentils
2-3 tablespoons olive oil
2 cups chicken broth
1 teaspoon sea salt
½ teaspoon freshly ground pepper

In skillet on stove top, sauté onion, garlic, cumin, and lentils in olive oil over medium heat for 10 minutes.

Add chicken broth, salt, and pepper, and simmer for 20-30 minutes on low heat.

Taste lentils as they cook, to test for desired doneness. They should be softened, yet not reduced to mush. Check periodically throughout cooking time to observe level of liquid; add water if needed.

Drain any extra water when finished; serve hot.

Makes 4 Servings

NUTRITIONAL FACTS

Serving Size 1/3 Cup Cooked

Amount per serving:

Calories 161

Total Fat 7.3g

Total Carbohydrate 17.6g

Dietary Fiber 6g

Sugars 2g

Protein 7.4g

VEGETABLE STIR FRY

We make the most of fresh garden produce by using in season vegetables in this recipe.

1 tablespoon fresh garlic, minced
2 tablespoons olive oil
1 cup broccoli florets
1 cup cauliflower
1 red pepper
1 green pepper
1 cup water chestnuts
½ small onion
1 carrot
1 zucchini
1 yellow summer squash
6-8 fresh mushrooms
Sea salt and freshly ground pepper
Chili powder or cayenne pepper, optional

Chop all veggies into 2" pieces. In large skillet on stove top, sauté minced garlic in olive oil for 3-5 minutes. Add vegetables. Sprinkle with salt, pepper, and other seasonings, if desired.

Stir fry over medium heat until vegetables are tender crisp. Serve immediately.

Makes 6 Servings

NUTRITIONAL FACTS

Serving Size 1 Cup

Amount per serving:

Calories 88

Total Fat 4.8g

Total Carbohydrate 8.2g

Dietary Fiber 3g

Sugars 5g

Protein 2.3g

GRILLED VEGETABLE PACKETS

1 zucchini
1 yellow summer squash
1 red pepper
1 onion, thinly sliced
1 carrot
Olive oil or melted butter for basting
Sea salt, freshly ground pepper, and garlic salt

Cut veggies into 1" pieces. On a large piece of heavy duty foil, sprayed with nonstick cooking spray, place veggies in single layer. Spritz with olive oil or melted butter. Sprinkle with sea salt, pepper, and garlic salt.

With a second piece of foil, cover veggies and wrap ends tightly to form sealed packet. Place on grill rack over medium heat and grill for 15 minutes.

When veggies are tender, remove from heat and serve.

Makes 4 Servings

TIPS TO TRY

Grilled Vegetable Packets are awesome for campfire cooking as well. Grill packets over medium-hot coals for 40 minutes or until tender.

NUTRITIONAL FACTS

Serving Size 1 Cup

Amount per serving:

Calories 64

Total Fat 3.7g

Total Carbohydrate 7.5g

Dietary Fiber 2g

Sugars 4g

Protein 1.7g

GRILLED ASPARAGUS

6 spears asparagus
Olive oil for basting
Sea salt and freshly ground pepper
Garlic salt, optional

Preheat grill to medium high.

Place washed asparagus spears on baking sheet or plate. Spritz or brush with olive oil, then sprinkle with desired seasonings.

Place spears on grill and allow to cook for 10 minutes. With fork or grill tongs, turn to ungrilled side. Grill additional 10 minutes, or until spears are slightly blackened and medium tender.

Remove from grill and serve immediately.

Makes 2 Servings

Grilled Asparagus pictured on pg. 130.

NUTRITIONAL FACTS

Serving Size 3 Spears

Amount per serving:

Calories 70

Total Fat 6.9g

Total Carbohydrate 1.9g

Dietary Fiber 1g

Sugars 1g

Protein 1.1g

LITTLE CHEDDAR MEAT LOAVES

Definitely child friendly because of the size and ingredients, mini meat loaves are a favorite.

Sauce:
⅔ cup **Homemade Ketchup (see Index)**
¼ cup **DaVinci® Pancake Sugar Free Syrup**
1½ teaspoons prepared mustard
¼ teaspoon liquid smoke

1 pound ground beef
1 cup shredded cheddar cheese
1 egg, beaten lightly
¼ cup heavy whipping cream
¼ cup tomato juice
½ cup fine bread crumbs (see Index for Almond Meal Dinner Rolls and Bread Crumbs)
½ onion, finely chopped
1 teaspoon sea salt

Preheat oven to 325°. In small bowl, combine sauce ingredients with spoon; set aside.

In larger bowl, combine beef and all following ingredients. Mix gently.

Form into 4 small individual meat loaves. Place in well greased baking pan. Ladle sauce over meat loaves. Bake for 1½ hours.

Makes 4 Servings

NUTRITIONAL FACTS

Serving Size 1 Loaf

Amount per serving:

Calories 556

Total Fat 41.5g

Total Carbohydrate 12.0g

Dietary Fiber 4g

Sugars 5g

Protein 34.8g

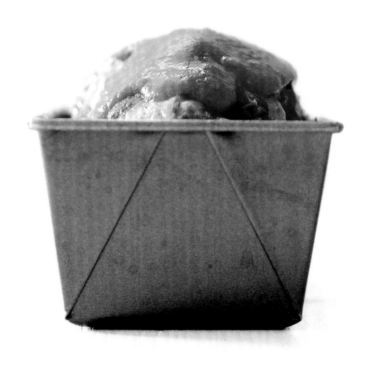

MEXICAN LASAGNA

This comfort food is a great replacement for classic lasagna.

1 tablespoon olive oil
1 small onion, finely chopped
1 pound ground beef
1 cup cooked pinto or kidney beans
2 tablespoons chili powder
4 low carb 8" tortillas, cut into 2" squares with kitchen shears
1 cup shredded cheddar cheese
2 cups Sugar Free Pizza Sauce (see Index)

Preheat oven to 350°. In large skillet, brown onion and beef in oil. When meat is no longer pink, add beans and chili powder. Cook for 4 minutes, stirring occasionally.

In greased 9" baking pan, place half of tortillas. Spoon beef mixture on top, and finish with remaining tortillas. Sprinkle with cheese and top with Sugar Free Pizza Sauce.

Bake for 1 hour or until heated through.

Makes 6 Servings (3" Squares)

NUTRITIONAL FACTS

Serving Size 1 Square
Amount per serving:
Calories 411
Total Fat 23.2g
Total Carbohydrate 23.2g
Dietary Fiber 9g
Sugars 6g
Protein 25.6g

BURRITO CASSEROLE

2 tablespoons cream cheese, softened
2 tablespoons sour cream
2 tablespoons water
¼ teaspoon cumin
½ teaspoon sea salt
¼ teaspoon freshly ground pepper
2 cups cooked chicken, cubed
4 low carb 8" tortillas

Your choice of topping from below:
½ cup Cheese Sauce (see Index)
½ cup Sugar Free Pizza Sauce (see Index)
½ cup Condensed Mushroom Soup (see Index) diluted with
2 tablespoons cream and 2 tablespoons water
½ cup shredded mozzarella or cheddar cheese

Preheat oven to 350°.

In small mixer bowl, blend cream cheese, sour cream, water, cumin, salt, and pepper. Gently stir in chicken.

Fill each tortilla with approximately 1/2 cup chicken filling, spread down center of tortilla. Roll up and place in greased 9" square baking pan.

Choose your topping, then sprinkle with cheese. Bake for 30 minutes.

Makes 4 Servings

NUTRITIONAL FACTS

Serving Size 1 Tortilla

Amount per serving:

Calories 384

Total Fat 20.6g

Total Carbohydrate 21.3g

Dietary Fiber 10g

Sugars 4g

Protein 25.0g

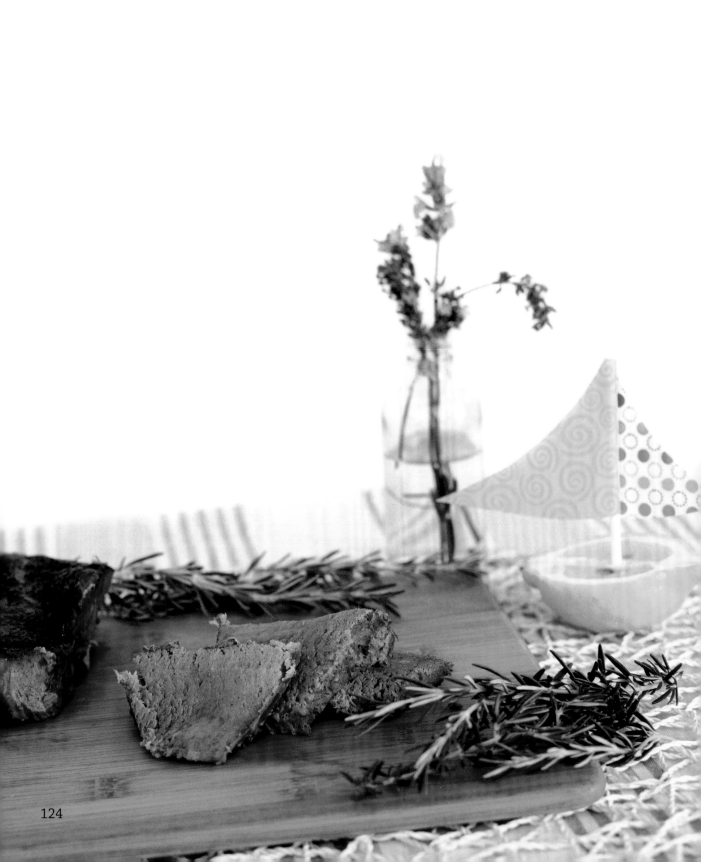

SLOW COOKER ROAST BEEF

A tried and true favorite, I save this dish for especially busy days.

1-2½ pounds beef roast
1 onion, thinly sliced
Sea salt and freshly ground pepper

Place frozen roast beef in slow cooker and add 2–3 inches of hot water. Spread onion on top of roast and sprinkle liberally with salt and pepper.

Cook on high for 3 hours, then reduce temperature to low and cook for additional 6 hours.

Makes 6 Servings

TIPS TO TRY

Adding carrots, zucchini, mushrooms, and summer squash halfway through the cooking time makes a great one dish meal for the whole family. To do this, prepare vegetables for cooking, then remove roast beef from slow cooker after the first 3 hours. Place veggies in bottom of slow cooker, sprinkle liberally with salt and pepper, and place roast beef on top. Cook an additional 6 hours as directed.

NUTRITIONAL FACTS

Serving Size 4 Ounces
Amount per serving:
Calories 114
Total Fat 4.5g
Total Carbohydrate 2.5g
Dietary Fiber 0g
Sugars 1g
Protein 15.7g

SWEET & TANGY BARBECUED MEATBALLS

Barbecued meatballs are among my earliest cooking recollections as a young girl. This recipe was a Sunday dinner mainstay through my growing up years. Andria had been on the diet several months before I realized that barbecue sauce is mostly just a tomato product with lots of molasses or honey and liquid smoke. The DaVinci® Pancake Sugar Free Syrup has been an awesome stand in since that lightning moment, and Andria is once again enjoying barbecued meatballs.

1 pound ground beef
¼ cup heavy whipping cream
1 egg, beaten
⅓ cup fine bread crumbs (see Index for Almond Meal Dinner Rolls and Bread Crumbs)
¼ onion, finely chopped
¼ teaspoon garlic powder
½ teaspoon sea salt
½ teaspoon chili powder

Sauce:
½ cup Homemade Ketchup (see Index)
1 teaspoon prepared mustard
2 tablespoons DaVinci® Pancake Sugar Free Syrup
¼ teaspoon liquid smoke

Preheat oven to 350°. Combine all ingredients for meatballs and mix gently. Form meat into 1" balls and place in greased 9" square baking pan.

Combine sauce ingredients in small bowl and mix. Pour sauce over meatballs and cover loosely with foil. Bake for 1 hour or until meat is no longer pink in center.

Makes 5 Servings

NUTRITIONAL FACTS

Serving Size 3 Meatballs

Amount per serving:

Calories 317

Total Fat 23.4g

Total Carbohydrate 5.9g

Dietary Fiber 2g

Sugars 2g

Protein 20.8g

STEAKS WITH SAUCE

A great recipe for less expensive cuts of steaks because the vinegar and lemon juice act as a tenderizer throughout the extended cooking time. Dine in tonight instead of dining out.

2 (12 ounce) sirloin or T-bone steaks or cut of choice
½ onion, finely chopped
2 tablespoons vinegar
1 tablespoon lemon juice
½ teaspoon sea salt
½ teaspoon freshly ground pepper
½ teaspoon dry mustard
¼ teaspoon garlic powder
½ cup Condensed Mushroom Soup (see Index)

Preheat oven to 225°. Place steaks in single layer in large, shallow baking pan. In small bowl, combine all following ingredients and pour over steaks. Bake for 4 hours.

Makes 4 Servings

TIPS TO TRY

Slow cooker method: Spray slow cooker with nonstick cooking spray. In small bowl, combine all ingredients (except steaks) and mix well. Place 1 steak in slow cooker. Cover with half of sauce. Repeat with remaining steak and sauce. Cook on high for 3 hours, and then on low 4 additional hours.

NUTRITIONAL FACTS

Serving Size 6 Ounces	
Amount per serving:	
Calories 455	
Total Fat 19.6g	
Total Carbohydrate 7.5g	
Dietary Fiber 2g	
Sugars 2g	
Protein 58.9g	

GRILLED FISH

2 (5 ounce) fish fillets of choice
1 teaspoon olive oil
Sea salt and freshly ground pepper, to taste
Juice of ½ lemon

Preheat broiler or outdoor grill. Rub the fillets with oil, then place under broiler (about 4 inches from heat source) or on grill. Cook for 4 minutes on each side, or until fish flakes easily with fork.

Season with salt, pepper, and lemon juice before serving.

Makes 2 Servings

TIPS TO TRY

To give the fillets a punch of extra flavor, combine equal parts olive oil and lemon juice with 1 clove crushed garlic. Brush on fish just before removing from grill.

NUTRITIONAL FACTS

Serving Size 1 Fish Fillet	
Amount per serving:	
Calories 119	
Total Fat 4g	
Total Carbohydrate 0.9g	
Dietary Fiber 0g	
Sugars 0g	
Protein 20.2g	

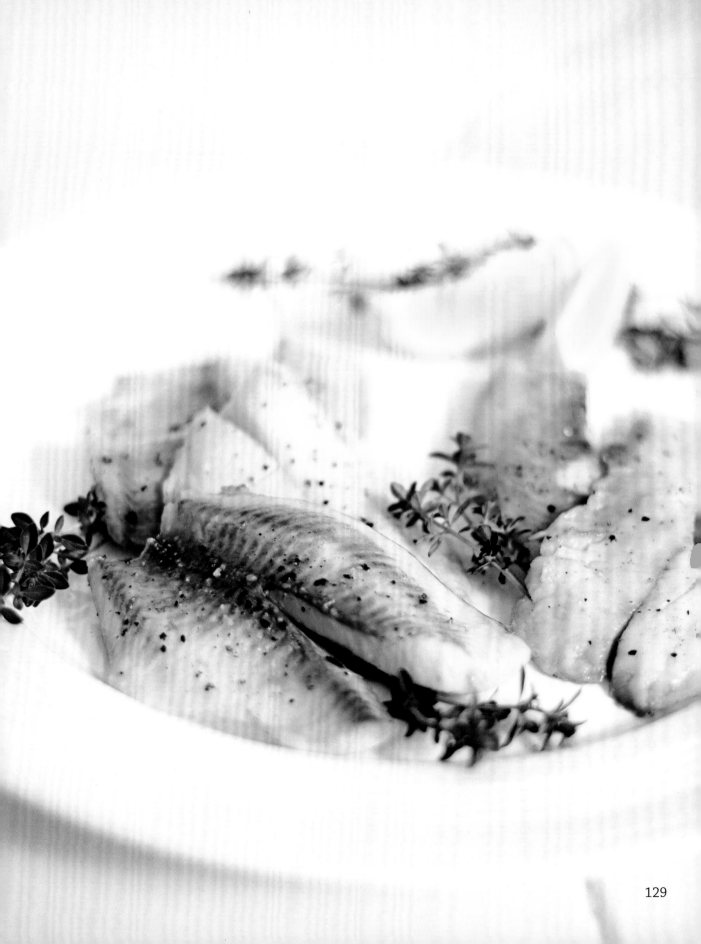

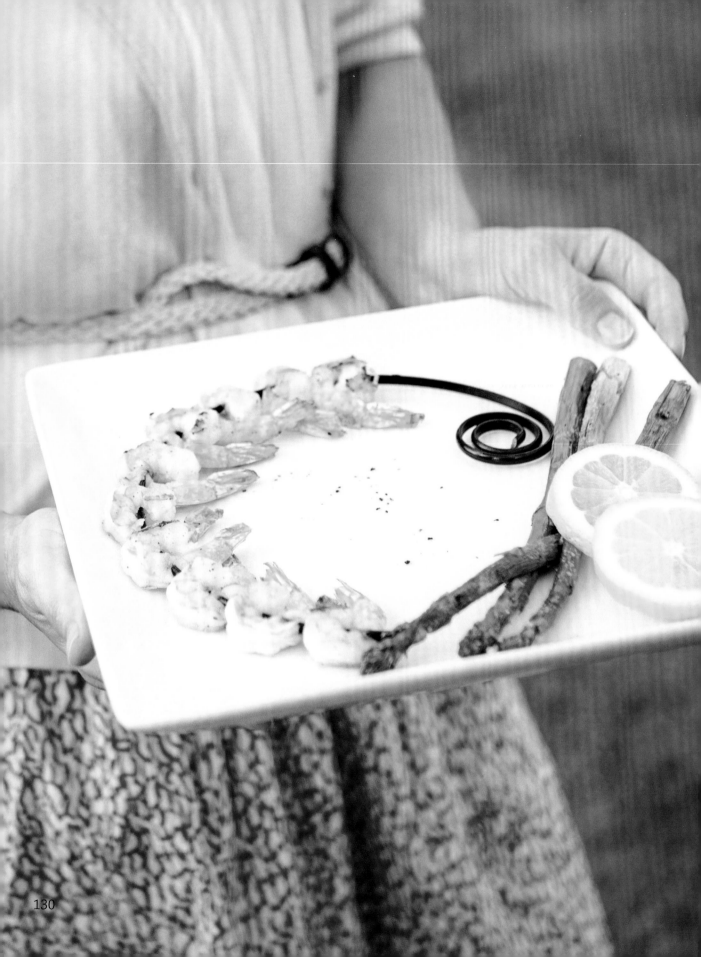

GRILLED SHRIMP SCAMPI

We are definitely grill fans, thanks to my husband. If I ask what he would like for dinner, he will invariably offer to grill. What a great trade off for my part of simply getting the meat in marinade!

2 tablespoons olive oil
2 tablespoons lemon juice
2 garlic cloves, minced
¼ teaspoon sea salt
¼ teaspoon freshly ground pepper
1½ pounds jumbo shrimp, peeled and deveined

In large bowl, whisk the first 5 ingredients. Add shrimp; toss to coat. Refrigerate, covered, for 30 minutes.

Thread shrimp onto 6 metal or wooden skewers soaked in water.

Grill, covered, over medium heat, or broil 4 inches from heat 6-8 minutes or until shrimp turn pink, turning once.

Makes 6 Servings

NUTRITIONAL FACTS

Serving Size 5-6 Shrimp

Amount per serving:

Calories 123

Total Fat 5.7g

Total Carbohydrate 1.7g

Dietary Fiber 0g

Sugars 0g

Protein 15.5g

OVEN BROILED FISH

My family loves this dish because it's delicious, and I love it because it's so easy. What a great catch!

4 fish fillets of choice (whiting, catfish, etc.)
4-6 tablespoons melted butter
Sea salt and freshly ground pepper

Preheat oven broiler. Spray shallow baking pan with nonstick cooking spray. Brush both sides of fillets with melted butter and sprinkle liberally with salt and pepper.

Broil 2-3 inches from broiler for 5-8 minutes.

Baste with melted butter, and return to oven for additional 5 minutes or until fish flakes easily with fork.

Makes 4 Servings

TIPS TO TRY

For a grilled version, brush fillets with olive oil and sprinkle with lemon pepper seasoning. Grill over medium heat until fish flakes easily with fork.

NUTRITIONAL FACTS

Serving Size 1 Fish Fillet
Amount per serving:
Calories 185
Total Fat 132.5g
Total Carbohydrate 0g
Dietary Fiber 0g
Sugars 0g
Protein 17.0g

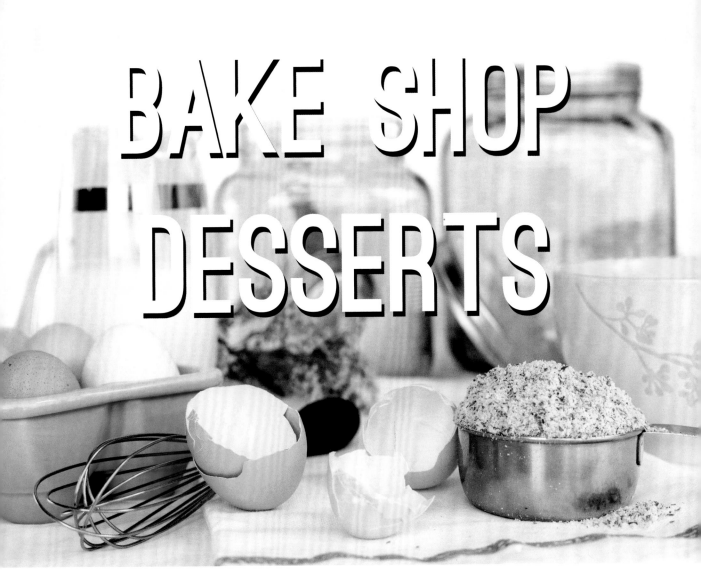

BAKE SHOP DESSERTS

sweet stuff

Move over, veggies and good for you fare! Make way for the parade of sweet stuff!
Welcome back, elegant cheesecake, parfait dishes, freshly baked cookies, and chocolate everything! Here at last I am truly at home. The grand finale at the end of a home cooked meal has always been my favorite part of food preparation.

As I relentlessly perused information, I found helpful and surprising knowledge on products I originally considered off limits. In the bakery line, probably the biggest change was portion size. Andria learned that a small treat was better than none at all.

My main sweetener in baking is stevia, and you will find a lot of cocoa in my collection. Cocoa makes it nearly impossible to taste the tiny bitterness of stevia.

Finding and developing these recipes has been the most fun and rewarding part of our cooking journey, because I had almost given up on ever serving dessert to Andria again!

"Sweets to the sweet!" - William Shakespeare

CHOCOLATE MOCHA COOKIES

¼ cup olive oil
¼ cup DaVinci® Pancake Sugar Free Syrup
4 drops liquid stevia
¾ cup plus 2 tablespoons almond meal
¼ cup sprouted wheat flour
2 tablespoons cocoa
1 tablespoon instant decaf coffee
¼ teaspoon baking soda
¼ teaspoon sea salt

Preheat oven to 350°. Combine olive oil, DaVinci® Pancake Sugar Free Syrup, and stevia. Mix well. Add almond meal, sprouted wheat flour, cocoa, instant coffee, baking soda, and sea salt. Blend until well combined. Shape dough into 12 small balls; flatten slightly.

Place on baking sheet. Bake for 10-12 minutes. Frost with Cream Cheese Frosting, or Cappuccino Frosting (see Index).

Makes 12 Servings

NUTRITIONAL FACTS *

Serving Size 1 Cookie

Amount per serving:

Calories 90

Total Fat 8.1g

Total Carbohydrate 3.9g

Dietary Fiber 1g

Sugars 0g

Protein 2.0g

Does not include frosting.

CHOCOLATE CHIP COOKIES

Return of a favorite in a mini version. Enjoy the classic, after school snack of a warm chocolate chip cookie.

¼ cup olive oil
¼ teaspoon liquid stevia
2 teaspoons pure vanilla extract
1 egg
1 tablespoon natural peanut butter
1 cup almond meal
¼ cup sprouted wheat flour
¼ teaspoon sea salt
¼ teaspoon baking soda
¼ cup Sugar Free Chocolate Chunks (see Index)

Preheat oven to 350°. Combine oil, stevia, vanilla, egg, and peanut butter. Mix well. Add almond meal, sprouted wheat flour, sea salt, and baking soda. Blend until well combined. Add chocolate chunks, stirring gently.

Shape dough into 15 small balls. Place on baking sheet and flatten slightly. Bake 10–12 minutes.

Makes 15 Servings

NUTRITIONAL FACTS

Serving Size 1 Cookie	
Amount per serving:	
Calories 108	
Total Fat 10.0g	
Total Carbohydrate 4.0g	
Dietary Fiber 2g	
Sugars 1g	
Protein 2.8g	

a bite
of happy

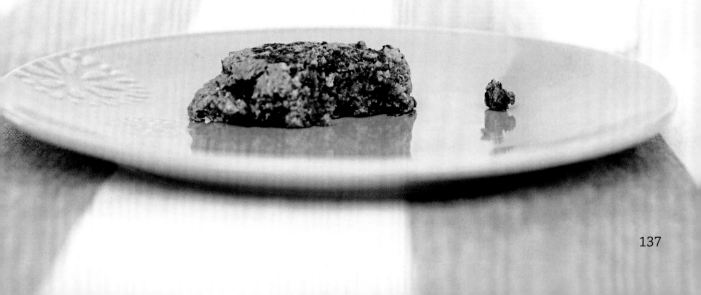

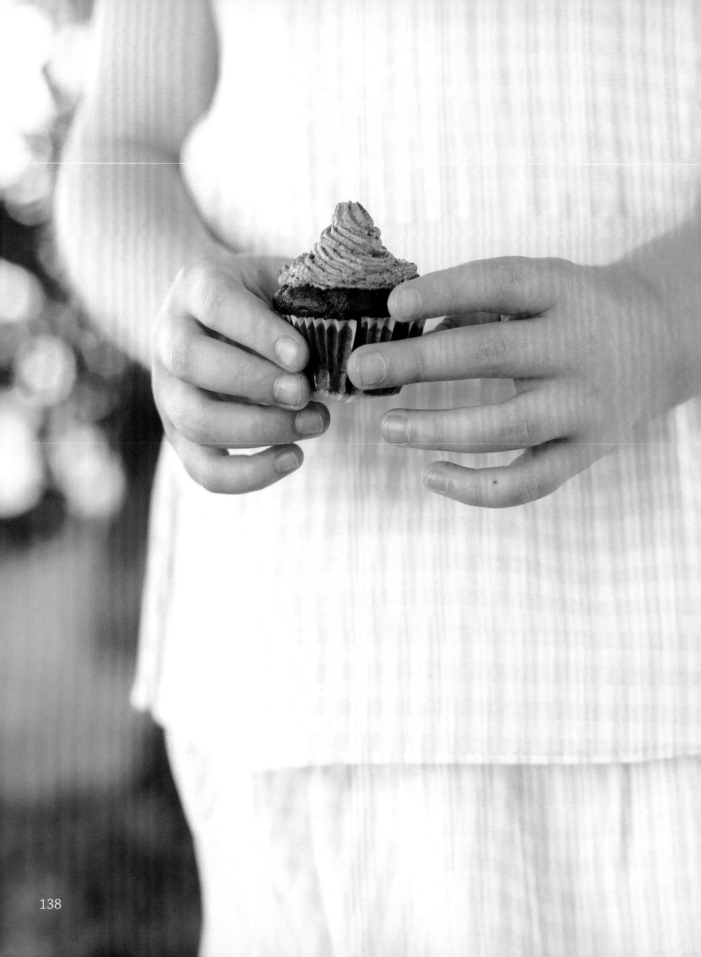

CAPPUCCINO MUFFINS

½ cup almond meal

2 tablespoons sprouted wheat flour

¼ teaspoon baking soda

⅛ teaspoon sea salt

2 tablespoons olive oil

⅛ teaspoon liquid stevia

1½ tablespoons DaVinci® Pancake Sugar Free Syrup

2 eggs

1 teaspoon pure vanilla extract

1 teaspoon instant decaf coffee

1 tablespoon cocoa

Preheat oven to 350°. Mix all ingredients and beat well.

Spoon into mini muffin liners, filling 3/4 full. Bake 8-12 minutes.

When cool, frost with Cappuccino or Cool Mint Frosting (see Index).

Makes 14 Servings

NUTRITIONAL FACTS

Serving Size 1 Mini Muffin

Amount per serving:

Calories 52

Total Fat 4.4g

Total Carbohydrate 1.8g

Dietary Fiber 1g

Sugars 0g

Protein 1.9g

GO PINK! CUPCAKES

This recipe was born from Andria's love of anything pink.

1 (15 oz.) can white kidney or navy beans
5 large eggs, plus 1 egg yolk
6 tablespoons butter, softened
⅛ teaspoon powdered stevia
1 tablespoon pure vanilla extract
6 tablespoons almond meal
½ teaspoon sea salt
½ teaspoon baking soda
1 teaspoon baking powder
8 drops red food coloring, optional
½ cup strawberries, coarsely chopped

Preheat oven to 350°. Rinse beans in cold water and drain well. Place in blender with eggs and egg yolk. Pulse on high until beans are smooth.

In bowl of stand mixer, cream butter until fluffy. Add stevia. Slowly add puréed bean/egg mixture, mixing on medium speed. Add remaining ingredients, except strawberries. Lightly fold berries into batter with spatula.

Spoon into mini cupcake liners, filling each one 3/4 full. Bake for 15-20 minutes, or until toothpick inserted in center comes out clean. Allow cupcakes to set for 24 hours to let the bean flavor disappear.

Makes 45 Servings

TIPS TO TRY

Frost with Go Pink! Frosting (see Index).

NUTRITIONAL FACTS

Serving Size 1 Mini Cupcake
Amount per serving:
Calories 40
Total Fat 2.7g
Total Carbohydrate 2.4g
Dietary Fiber 1g
Sugars 0g
Protein 1.1g

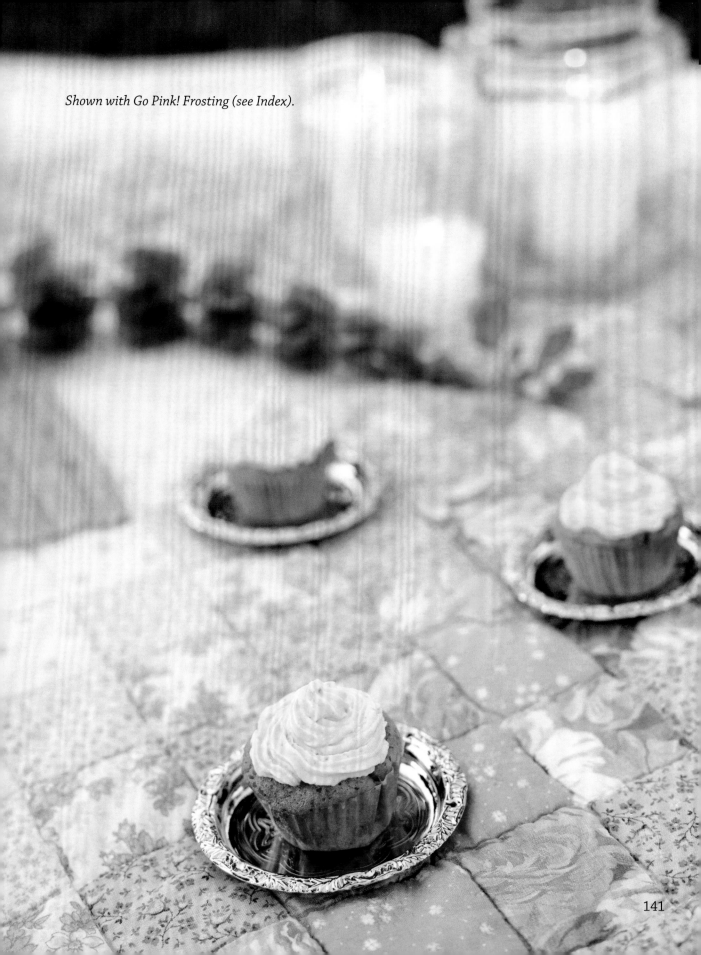

Shown with Go Pink! Frosting (see Index).

FUDGEY BROWNIES

Rich and chewy brownies show love anywhere, anytime. Keep a stash of almond butter on hand for a quick inspiration.

8 ounces creamy roasted almond butter

1 egg

½ cup DaVinci® Pancake Sugar Free Syrup

⅛ teaspoon powdered stevia

2 teaspoons pure vanilla extract

¼ cup cocoa

¼ teaspoon sea salt

½ teaspoon baking soda

Preheat oven to 350°. Combine almond butter, egg, DaVinci Pancake Sugar Free Syrup, stevia, and vanilla. Mix well. Add cocoa, sea salt, and baking soda. Blend until well combined and pour into greased 9" square baking pan.

Bake for 30-35 minutes or until toothpick inserted in center comes out clean.

Makes 16 Servings

NUTRITIONAL FACTS

Serving Size 1 Brownie
Amount per serving:
Calories 105
Total Fat 9.2g
Total Carbohydrate 3.8g
Dietary Fiber 2g
Sugars 1g
Protein 3.9g

POWER BARS

Attention! These bars are no bake. What could be easier, really?

1 cup raw almonds
¼ cup flaxseed meal
¼ cup unsweetened coconut
¼ cup creamy roasted almond butter
¼ teaspoon sea salt
¼ cup olive oil
2 drops liquid stevia
1 tablespoon DaVinci® Pancake Sugar Free Syrup
2 teaspoons pure vanilla extract

Place almonds, flaxseed meal, coconut, almond butter, and salt in food processor. Pulse briefly, about 10 seconds.

In small saucepan, combine olive oil, stevia, DaVinci® Pancake Sugar Free Syrup, and vanilla. Heat to simmering. Add to food processor and pulse until ingredients form a coarse paste.

Press into greased 8" glass square baking pan and refrigerate for 1 hour. Cut into squares and serve.

Makes 16 Servings

NUTRITIONAL FACTS

Serving Size 1 Bar

Amount per serving:

Calories 125

Total Fat 11.5g

Total Carbohydrate 4.1g

Dietary Fiber 2g

Sugars 1g

Protein 3.1g

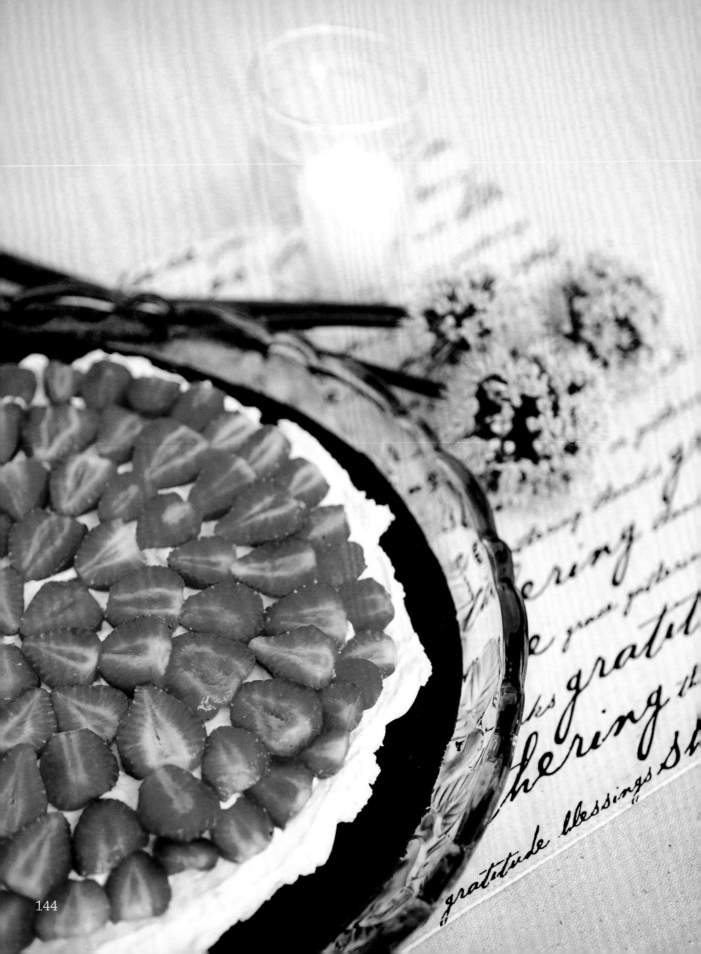

STRAWBERRY BROWNIE PIZZA

This brownie fruit pizza stars seasonal fresh fruit for an attractive summer dessert.

1 recipe Black Bean Brownies (see Index)
4 ounces cream cheese, softened
1 teaspoon pure vanilla extract
2½ tablespoons sugar free instant vanilla pudding (½ of a
1 oz. box)
2 cups Real Whipped Cream (see Index)
2 cups fresh strawberries
Additional Real Whipped Cream for garnish, optional

Preheat oven to 350°. Prepare brownies as directed in original recipe. Pour into greased medium pizza pan. Bake for 12–14 minutes or until toothpick inserted in center comes out clean. Cool.

In small bowl, beat cream cheese and vanilla until soft and creamy. Add pudding mix and beat well.

Gently add Real Whipped Cream. Do not overbeat. Spread over cooled brownie crust. Refrigerate.

Just before serving, top with fresh, sliced berries. Garnish with additional Real Whipped Cream if desired.

Makes 16 Servings

TIPS TO TRY

Any type of berry looks great on this dessert, or try a combination of 3 different berries.

NUTRITIONAL FACTS

Serving Size Per Wedge
Amount per serving:
Calories 182
Total Fat 15.2g
Total Carbohydrate 8.3g
Dietary Fiber 3g
Sugars 1g
Protein 4.3g

145

DECADENT STRAWBERRY BROWNIE TRIFLE

Here is your classic showstopper. No one will guess this recipe is low glycemic, much less sugar free. For a smaller group, try making half the recipe, and serving in individual parfait dishes or on small plates.

1 recipe Fudgey Brownies, or Black Bean Brownies (see Index)
4 ounces cream cheese, softened
2½ tablespoons sugar free instant vanilla pudding (½ of a 1 oz. box)
3 cups Real Whipped Cream (see Index)
2 cups fresh strawberries
Additional fresh strawberries for garnish, optional
Additional Real Whipped Cream for garnish, optional

Bake brownies according to directions; set aside to cool.

Meanwhile, in small bowl, mix cream cheese until soft and creamy. Add instant pudding mix and beat well. Gently add Real Whipped Cream. Do not overbeat.

Cut brownies into 1" cubes. In trifle bowl, place 1/3 of brownies. Top with 1/3 of cream mixture and berries. Repeat 2 more times.

Garnish with additional Real Whipped Cream and strawberries if desired. Chill 2 or 3 hours before serving.

Makes 16 Servings

TIPS TO TRY

Optional serving suggestion: Cut brownies into 16 pieces. On individual plates, place 1 brownie. Top with a dollop of cream filling and a strawberry.

NUTRITIONAL FACTS

Serving Size 2/3 Cup or 1 Brownie
Amount per serving:
Calories 242
Total Fat 22.6g
Total Carbohydrate 7.5g
Dietary Fiber 2g
Sugars 2g
Protein 5.1g

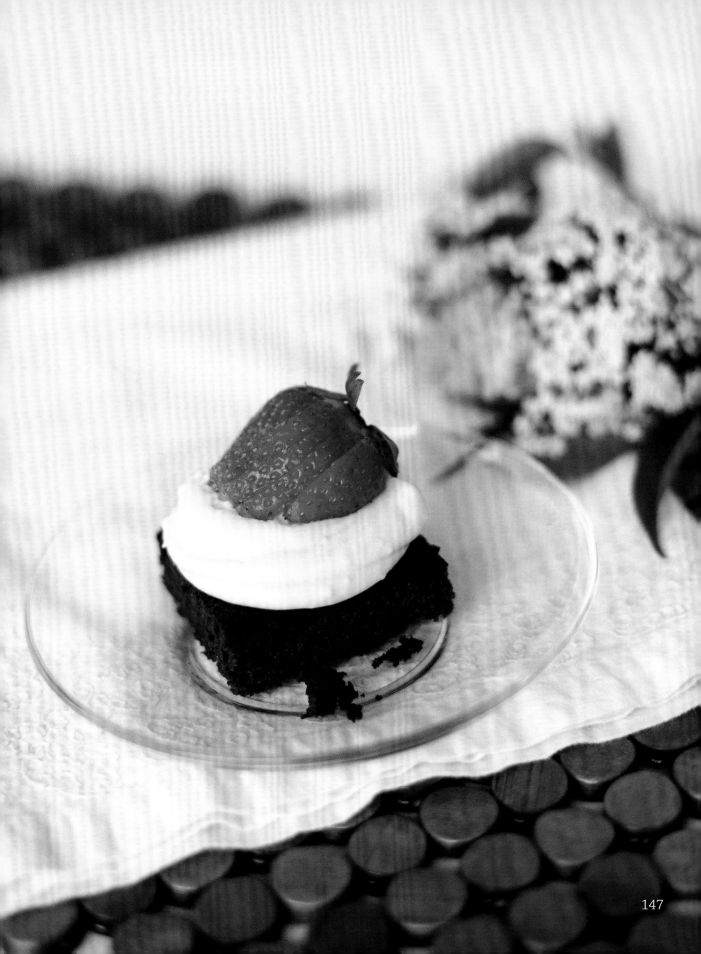

BLACK BEAN BROWNIES

Enter the era of healthy brownies. Chocolate cravings are cured fast in these chewy bites.

1½ cups cooked black beans, rinsed and drained
4 eggs
¼ teaspoon baking soda
½ teaspoon baking powder
3 tablespoons butter, melted
2 tablespoons oil
⅓ cup cocoa
¼ teaspoon sea salt
2 teaspoons pure vanilla extract
1 dash cayenne pepper
¼ teaspoon liquid stevia

Preheat oven to 350°. Place beans and eggs in blender and pulse until beans are totally smooth. Pour into mixing bowl and add remaining ingredients. Mix well.

Pour into greased 9" square baking pan. Bake for 20-25 minutes or until toothpick inserted in center comes out clean.

Makes 16 Servings

TIPS TO TRY

Let the brownies sit for 24 hours to allow the bean flavor to disappear. For a fun twist, frost brownies with Cool Mint Frosting or Cappuccino Frosting (see Index). Just remember to count the additional carbs.

NUTRITIONAL FACTS

Serving Size 1 Brownie
Amount per serving:
Calories 79
Total Fat 5.4g
Total Carbohydrate 5.0g
Dietary Fiber 2g
Sugars 0g
Protein 3.3g

DREAMSICLE JELL-O® CUPS

Dreamy. Creamy. This gelatin is delectable no matter what flavor you choose. Serving this in individual cups makes portion control easy.

1 cup boiling water
1 (0.3 oz.) box sugar free gelatin, any flavor
½ cup cold water
1 cup Real Whipped Cream (see Index)
2 ounces cream cheese, softened

Combine boiling water and gelatin. Stir until dissolved. Add cold water. Refrigerate until gelatin is beginning to set.

Place Real Whipped Cream in mixer bowl. Slowly add cream cheese in small pieces, blending after each addition.

Pour partially thickened gelatin into cream mixture in mixer bowl. Mix on low until well combined.

Pour into individual parfait dishes.

Makes 8 Servings

NUTRITIONAL FACTS

Serving Size 1/3 Cup	
Amount per serving:	
Calories 98	
Total Fat 9.8g	
Total Carbohydrate 1.5g	
Dietary Fiber 0g	
Sugars 0g	
Protein 1.5g	

VANILLA PUDDING

2½ tablespoons sugar free instant vanilla pudding (½ of a 1 oz. box)
½ cup heavy whipping cream
½ cup cold water
1½ cups Real Whipped Cream (see Index)

In 2 quart mixing bowl, combine 2½ tablespoons vanilla pudding mix, heavy whipping cream, and cold water. With mixer on low speed, beat for 2 minutes. Allow pudding mixture to soft set for 5 minutes in refrigerator.

Add Real Whipped Cream, stirring gently until well combined. Refrigerate until thoroughly chilled.

Makes 3 Servings

TIPS TO TRY

Use any flavor sugar free pudding that you enjoy.

NUTRITIONAL FACTS

Serving Size 3/4 Cup	
Amount per serving:	
Calories 427	
Total Fat 44.0g	
Total Carbohydrate 7.5g	
Dietary Fiber 0g	
Sugars 0g	
Protein 2.4g	

MANDARIN ORANGE PUDDING

I stumbled upon this recipe quite by accident. It caught my eye because the pudding is prepared with water instead of milk. Try it for a cool, creamy, summertime dessert.

2¼ cups hot water
1 (0.3 oz.) package sugar free orange gelatin
1 (0.8 oz.) sugar free cook style vanilla pudding
½ cup Skinny Libby® mandarin oranges, drained
2 cups Real Whipped Cream (see Index)

Place water, gelatin, and vanilla pudding in small saucepan. Bring to boil, then reduce heat and simmer for 5 minutes, stirring constantly.

Remove from heat and cool. Refrigerate until cold; 4-6 hours or overnight.

Just before serving, gently stir in oranges and Real Whipped Cream.

Makes 8 Servings

TIPS TO TRY

Variation—swap out the orange gelatin for strawberry and use fresh, sliced strawberries instead of mandarin oranges. Result: a lovely pink fluffy dessert! Serve in individual, stemmed parfait glasses, and garnish with additional Real Whipped Cream and a berry.

NUTRITIONAL FACTS

Serving Size 1/2 Cup
Amount per serving:
Calories 156
Total Fat 14.7g
Total Carbohydrate 5.5g
Dietary Fiber 0g
Sugars 1g
Protein 1.6g

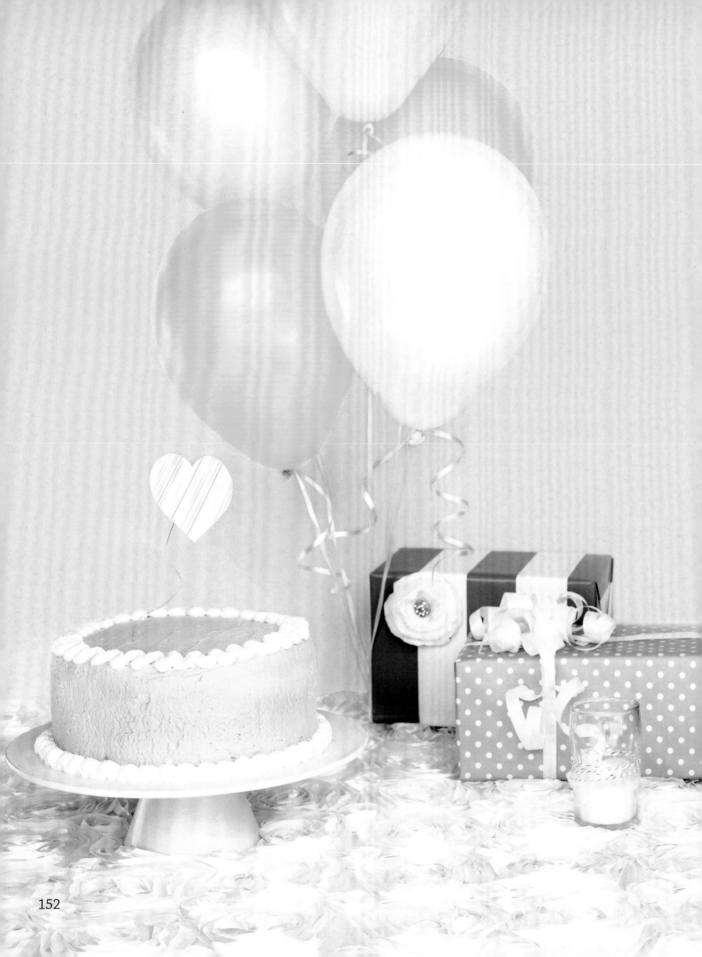

BLACK BEAN FUDGE CAKE

This was Andria's birthday cake the first year she was on the diet. Frosted with pink Real Whipped Cream (see Index), it looked like every little girl's dream cake. For a 2 layer cake, you will need 2 batches of batter. I recommend mixing 1 at a time.

1 (15 oz.) can black beans, rinsed and drained
5 large eggs, plus 1 egg white
1 teaspoon pure vanilla extract
½ teaspoon sea salt
6 tablespoons cocoa
1 teaspoon baking powder
½ teaspoon baking soda
6 tablespoons butter, softened
⅛ teaspoon powdered stevia
2 tablespoons sour cream

Preheat oven to 325°. Place beans, eggs and egg white, vanilla, and salt in blender or food processor. Blend on high until beans are liquefied.

In small bowl, whisk cocoa, soda, and baking powder.

In bowl of stand mixer, beat butter until light and fluffy. Add stevia and sour cream. Pour bean/egg mixture into bowl and mix. Add cocoa mixture and beat on high for 1 minute.

Grease or spray 8" round baking pan, then dust with cocoa. Pour batter into pan. Bake for 35-40 minutes, or until cake is round and firm. Cool.

Makes 16 Servings

TIPS TO TRY

This cake makes excellent cupcakes as well. Store in refrigerator for best flavor. Makes 24 cupcakes or 48 mini cupcakes.

NUTRITIONAL FACTS

Serving Size 1 Slice	
Amount per serving:	
Calories 94	
Total Fat 6.5g	
Total Carbohydrate 5.9g	
Dietary Fiber 3g	
Sugars 0g	
Protein 4.2g	

SUGAR FREE MOCHA CHEESECAKE

I was delighted to discover that the main ingredients in cheesecake are low glycemic. I use this mocha version the most because Andria loves anything with cocoa and coffee. For a vanilla version, simply skip the cocoa and coffee and serve with fresh fruit and Real Whipped Cream (see Index).

Crust:
½ cup almond meal
¼ cup pecans, ground
¼ cup sunflower seeds, ground
2 tablespoons butter, melted
Pinch of sea salt

Cheesecake:
2 (8 oz.) cream cheese bars, softened
3 eggs
⅛ teaspoon powdered stevia
1 teaspoon pure vanilla extract
1½ cups sour cream
1½ tablespoons instant coffee
2 tablespoons DaVinci® Chocolate Sugar Free Syrup

Topping:
⅓ cup heavy whipping cream
1 tablespoon butter, softened
2 ounces cream cheese, softened

Preheat oven to 325°. Prepare crust and press into a 9" round glass pan or an 8" springform pan.

In mixer bowl, beat cream cheese until soft and creamy. Add eggs 1 at a time, beating after each addition. Add all other ingredients, mixing on medium speed. Pour filling over crust and bake for 50 minutes or until filling is set.

For Topping: Using hand mixer, whip cream until soft peaks form. In separate bowl, mix butter and cream cheese until soft and creamy. Add cream cheese mixture to whipped cream slowly, 2 tablespoons at a time. Pipe onto cooled cheesecake just before serving. Dust with cocoa powder or drizzle with melted Sugar Free Chocolate Chunks (see index).

Makes 12 Servings

TIPS TO TRY

Begin by bringing all ingredients to room temperature.

Add eggs one at a time, and beat just until blended. Do not over mix.

No peeking! Keep the oven door closed during baking to prevent cheesecake from cracking.

NUTRITIONAL FACTS

Serving Size 1 Slice	
Amount per serving:	
Calories	333
Total Fat	32.2g
Total Carbohydrate	5.7g
Dietary Fiber	1g
Sugars	3g
Protein	6.8g

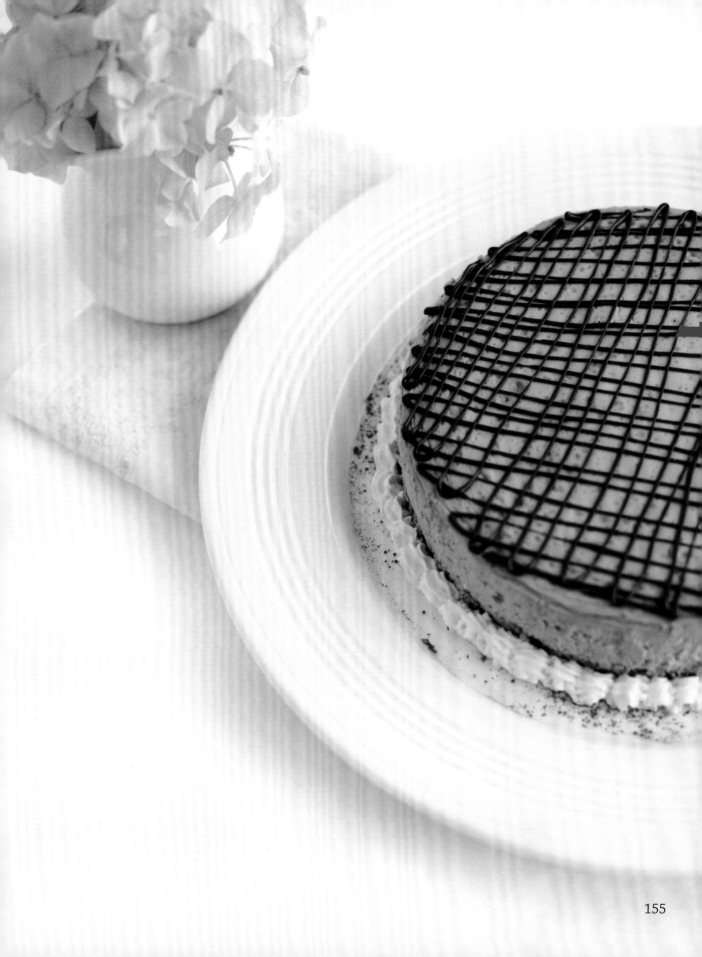

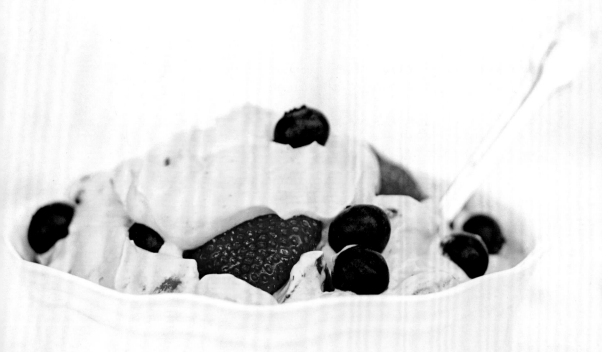

DREAMY FRUIT SALAD

The cream cheese in this dessert hides any of the low glycemic or sugar free taste. Use any combination of fresh berries that appeals to you.

1 cup Real Whipped Cream (see Index)
2 ounces cream cheese, softened
½ tablespoon lemon juice
½ cup low carb vanilla yogurt
4 cups fresh fruit (of choice)
  ½ cup chopped fresh strawberries
  ½ cup raspberries
  ½ cup blackberries
  ¼ cup chopped apples
  ¼ cup blueberries

Prepare Real Whipped Cream.

In separate bowl, beat cream cheese until smooth and creamy.
Add lemon juice and yogurt. Gently stir in Real Whipped Cream.

Just before serving, fold fruit into mixture. Serve chilled.

Makes 5 Servings

NUTRITIONAL FACTS

Serving Size 1 Cup
Amount per serving:
Calories 183
Total Fat 16.1g
Total Carbohydrate 8.4g
Dietary Fiber 2g
Sugars 4g
Protein 3.1g

REAL WHIPPED CREAM

This is one of my most used recipes. Use it in any gelatin or dessert recipe, as well as garnish for hot drinks or frothy shakes.

⅔ cup heavy whipping cream
20 drops liquid sucralose
3 teaspoons clear imitation vanilla flavoring

Begin by placing 2 quart mixing bowl, hand mixer beaters, and cream in freezer for 5 minutes.

Combine cream, sucralose, and vanilla in chilled bowl. With hand mixer on high speed, beat until stiff peaks form, approximately 1 minute and 30 seconds. (Decrease or increase time if you are doing less cream or a double batch at once.) Overbeating will cause cream to "fall" and lose its stiffness.

Makes 1 Serving

TIPS TO TRY

Although this cream can be done in a stand mixer with a wire beater, I have much more success using my hand mixer because I can judge better the stiffness of the cream and know when it reaches its optimum.

NUTRITIONAL FACTS

Serving Size 1 Cup	
Amount per serving:	
Calories 553	
Total Fat 58.6g	
Total Carbohydrate 6.2g	
Dietary Fiber 0g	
Sugars 0g	
Protein 3.2g	

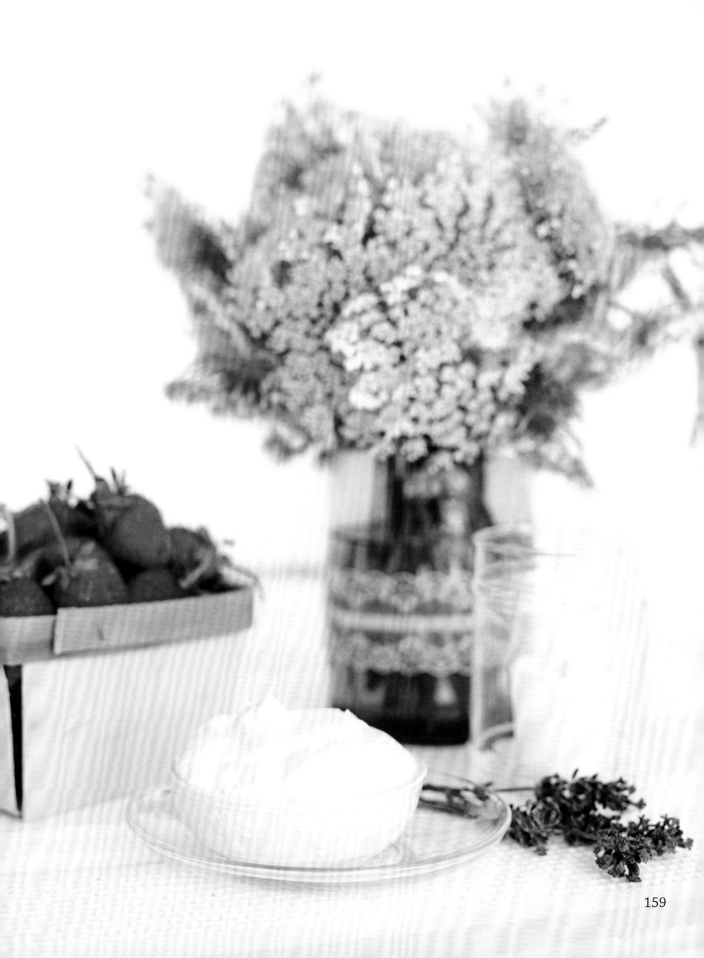

CREAM CHEESE FROSTING

Believe it or not, it's still okay to indulge your taste buds.

4 ounces cream cheese, softened
1 tablespoon butter, softened
4 drops liquid sucralose
½ teaspoon clear imitation vanilla flavoring
4 tablespoons Real Whipped Cream (see Index)

Beat cream cheese until creamy. Add softened butter, sucralose, and vanilla and mix well. Blend in Real Whipped Cream. Store in refrigerator.

Makes 26 Servings
Frosts approximately 26 mini cupcakes or cookies.

NUTRITIONAL FACTS

Serving Size 1/2 Tablespoon
Amount per serving:
Calories 24
Total Fat 2.5g
Total Carbohydrate 0.3g
Dietary Fiber 0g
Sugars 0g
Protein 0.3g

GO PINK! FROSTING

1½ cups Real Whipped Cream (see Index)
2 ounces cream cheese, softened
2 teaspoons sugar free strawberry gelatin

Prepare Real Whipped Cream.

In separate bowl, beat cream cheese and gelatin until creamy and smooth. Stir in Real Whipped Cream.

With large tip on cake decorator, pipe onto Go Pink! Cupcakes (see Index). Store in refrigerator.

Makes 45 Servings
Frosts 45 mini cupcakes.

Go Pink! Frosting pictured on pg. 141.

NUTRITIONAL FACTS

Serving Size 1/2 Tablespoon	
Amount per serving:	
Calories 23	
Total Fat 2.4g	
Total Carbohydrate 0.3g	
Dietary Fiber 0g	
Sugars 0g	
Protein 0.3g	

COOL MINT FROSTING

This recipe was inspired from mint chocolate chip cupcakes. Use as frosting on cappuccino muffins, to dress up brownies, or even on a birthday cake. A lovely presentation and change of pace.

½ cup Real Whipped Cream (see Index)
1 drop peppermint oil
1 drop green food coloring, optional
1 ounce cream cheese, softened and cut into chunks

Mix Real Whipped Cream according to instructions. Just before stiff peaks form, add peppermint oil, food coloring, and cream cheese.

Beat on low until well combined, but do not overbeat, as this will cause cream to "fall". Store in refrigerator.

Makes 15 Servings
Makes enough to frost 15 cappuccino muffins.

Cool Mint Frosting pictured on pg. 152.

NUTRITIONAL FACTS

Serving Size 1/2 Tablespoon	
Amount per serving:	
Calories 25	
Total Fat 2.6g	
Total Carbohydrate 0.3g	
Dietary Fiber 0g	
Sugars 0g	
Protein 0.2g	

CAPPUCCINO FROSTING

Delectable and irresistible! Use on brownies or muffins.

4 ounces cream cheese, softened
1 tablespoon cocoa
1 teaspoon instant decaf coffee
½ teaspoon pure vanilla extract
3 drops liquid stevia

Mix all ingredients until smooth. Store in refrigerator.

Makes 6 Servings
Makes enough to frost 6-8 brownies.

Cappuccino Frosting pictured on pg. 138.

NUTRITIONAL FACTS

Serving Size 1/2 Tablespoon
Amount per serving:
Calories 37
Total Fat 3.4g
Total Carbohydrate 1.2g
Dietary Fiber 0g
Sugars 0g
Protein 0.8g

CHOCOLATE MOUSSE

This mousse stands alone as a dessert in a parfait dish, or I use it as frosting for birthday cakes or cupcakes.

½ tablespoon unflavored gelatin
1 tablespoon cold water
3 tablespoons hot water
1 cup heavy whipping cream
¼ teaspoon liquid stevia
1 teaspoon pure vanilla extract
2 tablespoons cocoa

In small bowl, mix gelatin with cold water. Allow to rest for 5 minutes. Stir into hot water until dissolved; allow to cool slightly.

Beat cream in separate bowl until soft peaks form. Gently add gelatin mixture and remaining ingredients. Refrigerate.

Makes 6 Servings

NUTRITIONAL FACTS

Serving Size 1/4 Cup

Amount per serving:

Calories 145

Total Fat 14.9g

Total Carbohydrate 2.2g

Dietary Fiber 1g

Sugars 0g

Protein 1.7g

ELEGANT CHOCOLATE GLAZE

Perfect for garnishing desserts or a quick drizzle over lattés.

¼ cup heavy whipping cream
1 (6 oz.) bar unsweetened baking chocolate
1 tablespoon butter
½ teaspoon pure vanilla extract
8 drops liquid sucralose
⅛ teaspoon liquid stevia
Pinch of sea salt

In small saucepan, heat cream over medium heat until simmering, stirring constantly. Set aside. Break unsweetened chocolate into small pieces and place in food processor or blender with butter, vanilla, salt, sucralose, and stevia.

Pour hot cream over mixture in blender and process until chocolate is melted and mixture is completely smooth. Drizzle over cakes, cookies, or cupcakes. Store in refrigerator.

Makes 8 Servings

TIPS TO TRY

The consistency of this glaze should be medium thick. If too thick, add a bit of hot water. If too thin, pop into fridge for 15 minutes, then re-blend.

NUTRITIONAL FACTS

Serving Size 1 Tablespoon
Amount per serving:
Calories 146
Total Fat 15.3g
Total Carbohydrate 6.6g
Dietary Fiber 4g
Sugars 0g
Protein 2.9g

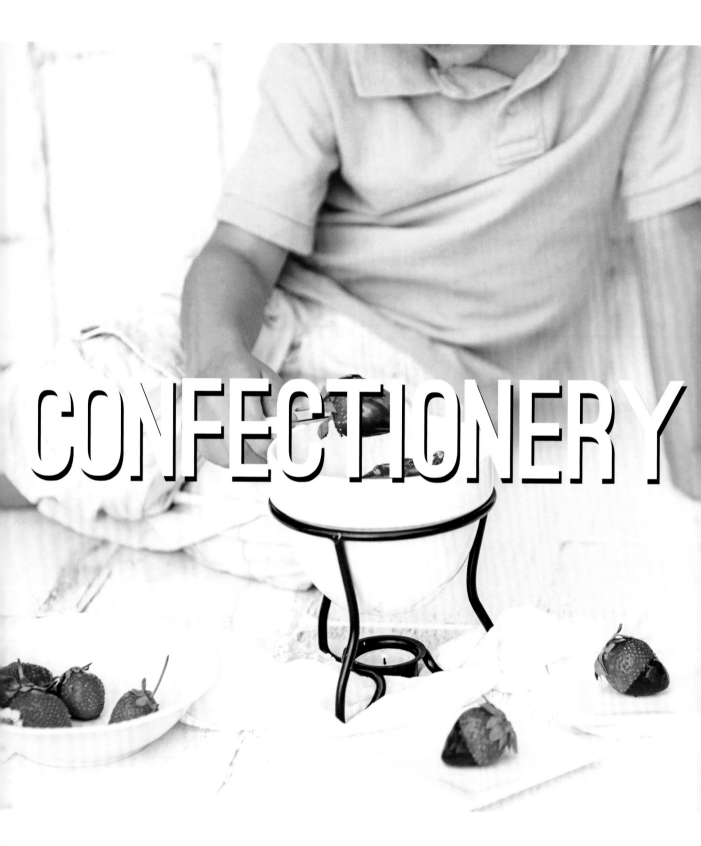

CONFECTIONERY

indulge a little

Here are the one bite indulgences that every person craves now and then, or needs a taste of just to make it through the day. Although this type of candy takes a bit more detailed attention, the result is a sugar free chocolate, with no high carb numbers from sugar alcohols. Pair dark chocolate with peanuts, macadamias, or pecans for a gourmet, low glycemic treat. These sweets are my own secret arsenal which I keep stashed in the freezer for weak moments, special days at school, or when the rest of the family is enjoying s'mores beside a campfire. Life is better with chocolate!

CHOCOLATE COVERED PEANUT CLUSTERS

Swap out the peanuts for almonds, pecans, walnuts, or macadamias.

6 tablespoons roasted, salted peanuts
2 tablespoons Sugar Free Chocolate Chunks (see Index)

Line baking sheet with parchment paper. Melt Sugar Free Chocolate Chunks in microwave according to recipe instructions. In small bowl, pour melted chocolate over peanuts, tossing to coat.

Drop by teaspoons onto parchment paper. Chill.

Makes 12 Servings

Chocolate Covered Peanut Clusters pictured on pg. 171.

NUTRITIONAL FACTS

Serving Size 1 Cluster	
Amount per serving:	
Calories 39	
Total Fat 3.7g	
Total Carbohydrate 1.4g	
Dietary Fiber 1g	
Sugars 0g	
Protein 1.5g	

DELUXE SUGAR FREE TRUFFLES

At last! A chocolate candy that I can stash in the freezer and pull out for special occasions or emergency moments.

1 (4 oz.) bar unsweetened baking chocolate
1½ tablespoons butter
¼ cup cream
2 teaspoons pure vanilla extract
8 drops liquid sucralose
⅛ teaspoon liquid stevia
pecans, finely chopped, optional
cocoa and cinnamon mixture, for dusting, optional

In small saucepan on stove top, heat all ingredients over low heat, stirring constantly until melted; blend well.

Chill in refrigerator until slightly hardened and easy to handle, approximately 2 hours. Form into 1" balls. Roll in chopped pecans, or cocoa and cinnamon.

Makes 18 Servings

Deluxe Sugar Free Truffles pictured on pg. 171.

NUTRITIONAL FACTS

Serving Size 1 Truffle	
Amount per serving:	
Calories 53	
Total Fat 5.5g	
Total Carbohydrate 2.0g	
Dietary Fiber 1g	
Sugars 0g	
Protein 0.9g	

SUGAR FREE BUCKEYE CANDIES

½ cup plus 2 tablespoons creamy natural peanut butter
¼ cup ricotta cheese
2 tablespoons butter, softened
¼ teaspoon pure vanilla extract
⅛ teaspoon powdered stevia
Pinch of sea salt
⅔ cup Sugar Free Chocolate Chunks (see Index); *equals 1 whole serving*

In food processor, combine first 6 ingredients. Spread in shallow pan and place in freezer until filling is firm enough to handle. Shape into 1" balls. Return to freezer for 1 hour.

Line a baking sheet with parchment paper. Melt Sugar Free Chocolate Chunks in microwave according to recipe instructions.

Using a toothpick to lift buckeye, dip in melted chocolate, leaving a small area at tip of candy for filling to peek through. Place on parchment lined baking sheet and refrigerate until firm.

Store in freezer or refrigerator.

Makes 30 Servings

NUTRITIONAL FACTS

Serving Size 1 Buckeye

Amount per serving:

Calories 53

Total Fat 4.9g

Total Carbohydrate 1.7g

Dietary Fiber 1g

Sugars 1g

Protein 1.8g

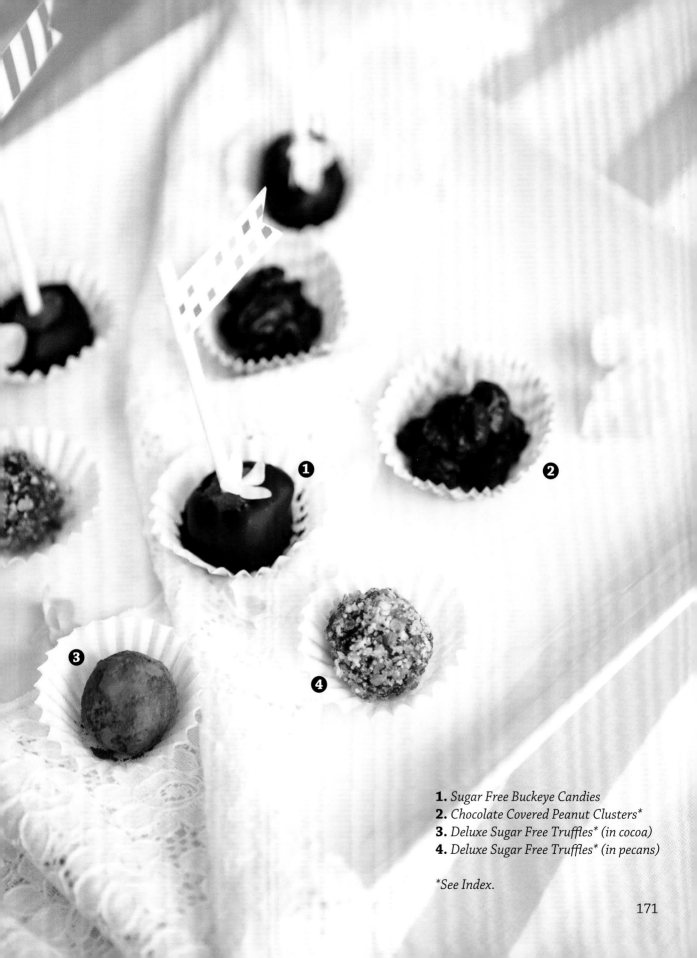

1. *Sugar Free Buckeye Candies*
2. *Chocolate Covered Peanut Clusters**
3. *Deluxe Sugar Free Truffles* (in cocoa)*
4. *Deluxe Sugar Free Truffles* (in pecans)*

See Index.

171

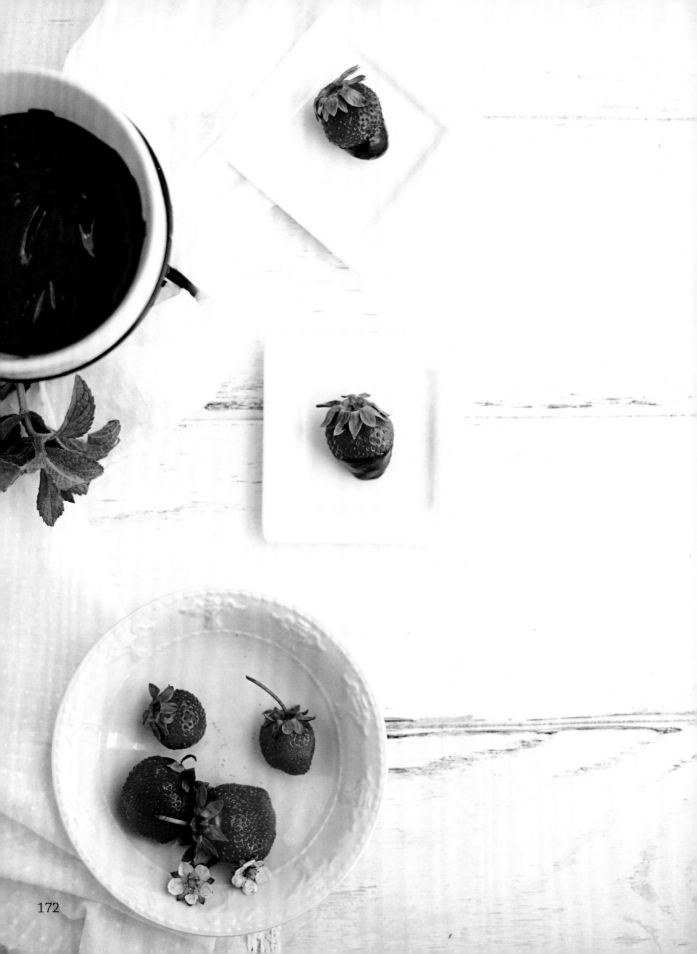

CHOCOLATE DIPPED STRAWBERRIES

6 fresh strawberries, washed
2 ounces Sugar Free Chocolate Chunks (see Index)

Melt Sugar Free Chocolate Chunks in microwave according to
recipe instructions.

Using a fondue fork, dip bottom half of berry in chocolate. Place
on waxed paper and allow chocolate to harden, or quick chill in
refrigerator.

Makes 6 Servings

NUTRITIONAL FACTS

Serving Size 1 Strawberry
Amount per serving:
Calories 58
Total Fat 5.7g
Total Carbohydrate 3.7g
Dietary Fiber 2g
Sugars 1g
Protein 1.3g

SUGAR FREE CHOCOLATE CHUNKS

This chocolate method can also be used with 85% or 90% cacao bars. Adjust sweetener to suit your taste.

2 ounces unsweetened baking chocolate
1 teaspoon shortening
6 drops liquid sucralose
1/16 teaspoon powdered stevia

In microwave safe bowl, heat all ingredients at 50% power for 1 minute. Stir. Continue heating and stirring in 20-30 second intervals until chocolate is smooth and totally melted.

Pour onto a 9" pan lined with parchment paper and spread. Allow to harden, then break or chop into small chunks.

Makes 1 Serving

TIPS TO TRY

Use this method and recipe to dip Deluxe Sugar Free Truffles* and to make Chocolate Covered Peanut Clusters*. Chocolate Chunks can easily be stored in freezer and remelted. I also chop these finely and use in Chocolate Chip Cookies*. Yum!

*(see Index)

NUTRITIONAL FACTS

Serving Size 2 Ounces
Amount per serving:
Calories 321
Total Fat 33.9g
Total Carbohydrate 16.9g
Dietary Fiber 9g
Sugars 1g
Protein 7.3g

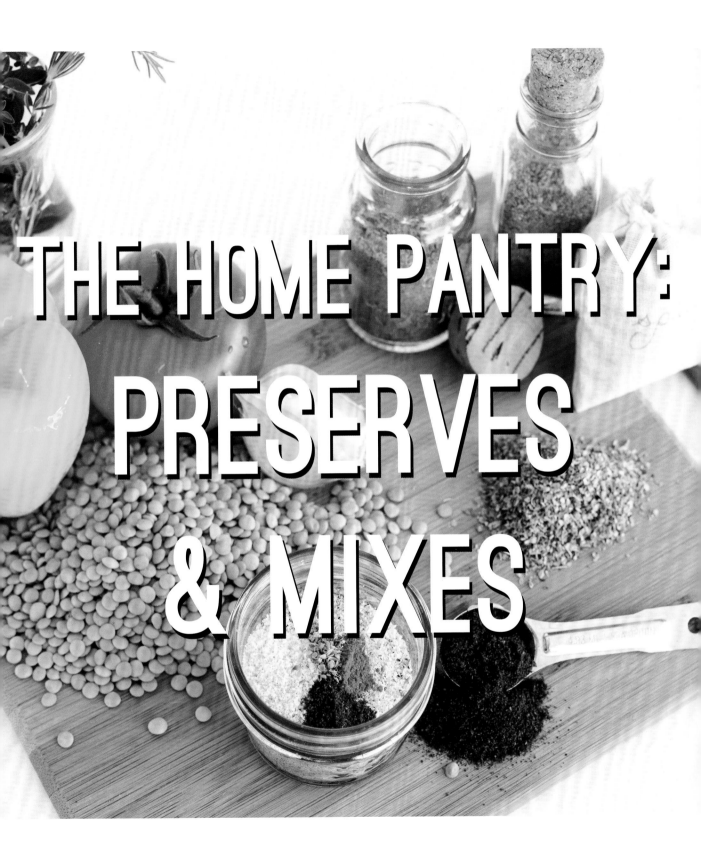

THE HOME PANTRY:
PRESERVES
& MIXES

mix it up

Although this section is brief, I can't imagine the diet without it. The good thing about the tomato based recipes is that you can choose between starting with fresh, ripe tomatoes, or the canned juice or purée. I have done both and found the taste to be better with fresh tomatoes, which makes good use of our fresh garden produce. The ketchup, especially, has become an essential in Andria's diet and is not difficult to make. The extra effort is well worth the variety it has added to her diet options.

The idea of creating seasoning mixes came with the beginning of my food label reading when I realized the lurking places of hidden carbs. The seasoning recipes here are extremely easy to make. Invest in glass or clear plastic shakers that can be labeled, and you are ready to cook!

CHEESE SAUCE

I like to make a batch of cheese sauce at the beginning of the week, then plan Andria's menus around the dishes that include it in the ingredients. Generally use only 2-4 tablespoons at a time.

4 ounces Velveeta® cheese
2 ounces cream cheese
4 tablespoons sour cream
2-3 tablespoons heavy whipping cream or water

In microwave safe bowl, combine first 3 ingredients. Heat for 1 minute at 50% power. Add water or cream, and heat an additional 30 seconds.

Blend with immersion blender until smooth. Add sea salt and freshly ground pepper to taste.

Makes 4 Servings

NUTRITIONAL FACTS

Serving Size 1/4 Cup	
Amount per serving:	
Calories 157	
Total Fat 13.4g	
Total Carbohydrate 3.7g	
Dietary Fiber 0g	
Sugars 3g	
Protein 5.7g	

HOMEMADE KETCHUP

This recipe is another in my list of lifesavers. Plan on several hours for the cooking and simmering process, although the ketchup does not require constant stirring. For easy use, buy a squeeze bottle to keep in the refrigerator.

4 quarts tomato juice or 1 (6 lb. 10 oz.) can tomato sauce
1 cup apple cider vinegar
¾ teaspoon powdered stevia
¼ cup sea salt
1 onion, puréed
⅓ teaspoon cinnamon
⅓ teaspoon ginger
⅓ teaspoon cloves
⅓ teaspoon nutmeg
3 (12 oz.) cans tomato paste

If using tomato juice, pour into large kettle or stock pot and bring to a boil. Reduce heat and allow to simmer, uncovered, until water evaporates, leaving liquid at about half the original level.

If beginning with tomato sauce, eliminate the first step, and pour sauce and all ingredients (except tomato paste) into large, heavy kettle. Bring to boil, then reduce heat and simmer for 35 minutes, stirring occasionally. Add tomato paste and bring to boil again.

Remove from heat and ladle into 1 cup glass jars. To preserve, can with water bath method or freeze. Ketchup can be stored in refrigerator for several weeks.

Makes 256 Servings (16 cups)

TIPS TO TRY

Although this will taste a bit different from commercial brands of ketchup, Andria loved it after she made the initial change. This opened the door to cheeseburgers and an occasional hotdog again—without the bun, of course.

NUTRITIONAL FACTS

Serving Size 1 Tablespoon	
Amount per serving:	
Calories 6	
Total Fat 0g	
Total Carbohydrate 1.4g	
Dietary Fiber 0g	
Sugars 1g	
Protein 0.3g	

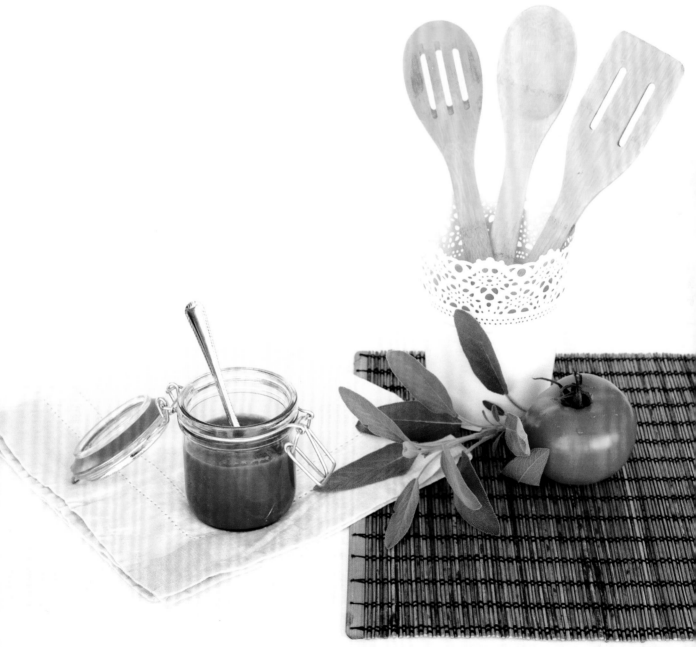

SALSA OLÉ

We have been eating homemade salsa for so long we have lost our taste for commercially canned salsa! This recipe pulls together all the flavors into one delicious, spicy blend. Serve with tortilla pinwheels or any type of wrap.

1 onion
2 cloves garlic
¼ cup jalapeños, canned or fresh
1 green pepper
12 cups peeled, chopped tomatoes, drained
¼ teaspoon powdered stevia
¾ cup apple cider vinegar
1 tablespoon dried cilantro
1 teaspoon parsley
2 teaspoons sea salt
⅛ teaspoon cayenne pepper
⅛ teaspoon freshly ground pepper
⅛ teaspoon paprika
⅛ teaspoon cumin
1 teaspoon citric acid, optional

In mini chopper, combine onion, garlic, jalapeños, and green pepper, pulsing until chopped fine.

Mix with all other ingredients in large heavy kettle. Bring to boil, then reduce heat and simmer for 1 hour, stirring occasionally to keep from scorching.

Ladle into jars or containers. To preserve: can with the water bath method, or freeze.

Makes 64 Servings (16 cups)

NUTRITIONAL FACTS

Serving Size 1/4 Cup	
Amount per serving:	
Calories 5	
Total Fat 0g	
Total Carbohydrate 0.9g	
Dietary Fiber 0g	
Sugars 1g	
Protein 0.2g	

SUGAR FREE PIZZA SAUCE

4½ quarts tomato juice or 1 (6 lb. 10 oz.) can tomato sauce
2 tablespoons garlic
2 medium onions, puréed
¾ cup olive oil
2 (12 oz.) cans tomato paste
1½ tablespoons basil
1½ tablespoons oregano
½ teaspoon powdered stevia
2 tablespoons sea salt

If using tomato juice, pour into large, heavy kettle or stock pot. Bring to boil, lower temperature, and allow to simmer with kettle uncovered until juice level reaches half its original volume.

If using tomato sauce, eliminate the first step, and pour all ingredients into large kettle. Bring to boil, then simmer for 30 minutes, stirring occasionally to keep from scorching.

Ladle into glass jars or containers. To preserve, can with the water bath method, or freeze.

Makes 36 Servings (18 cups)

TIPS TO TRY

This is my "everything" sauce. I use it for sloppy joes, taco salad, pizza burgers, and as a sauce for baked enchiladas.

NUTRITIONAL FACTS

Serving Size 1/2 Cup	
Amount per serving:	
Calories 79	
Total Fat 4.7g	
Total Carbohydrate 9.3g	
Dietary Fiber 1g	
Sugars 7g	
Protein 1.8g	

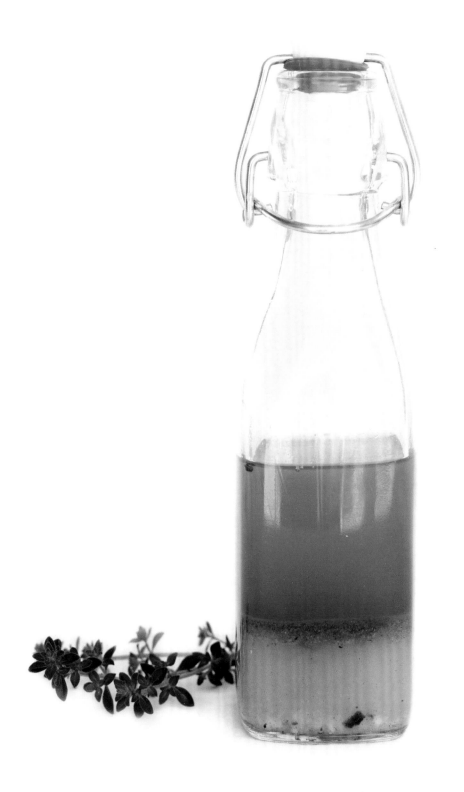

HERBED CHICKEN MARINADE

½ cup olive oil
1 garlic clove, minced
1 teaspoon ground sage
½ cup lemon juice
1½ teaspoons rosemary
¼ teaspoon freshly ground pepper

Combine all marinade ingredients.

Makes 4 Servings

TIPS TO TRY

This marinade creates a succulent, savory main dish of poultry or steak. Pour over meat of choice and marinate in refrigerator 6 hours or overnight.

NUTRITIONAL FACTS

Serving Size 1/4 Cup

Amount per serving:

Calories 247

Total Fat 27.1g

Total Carbohydrate 2.4g

Dietary Fiber 0g

Sugars 1g

Protein 0g

SEASONED SALT

1 cup Real Salt® or sea salt
2 tablespoons onion powder
1 teaspoon garlic powder
1 tablespoon celery salt
2 teaspoons paprika
1 teaspoon chili powder
1 teaspoon parsley flakes

Blend all ingredients in small bowl with a fork or spoon. Store in tightly closed glass jar or spice shaker. Use on grilled meats, fish, or eggs.

Makes 1¼ Cups

NUTRITIONAL FACTS

*This is considered a **free food** as the carbs are low enough to remain uncalculated.*

FAJITA SEASONING

Fajita Seasoning is my favorite blend of spices for preparing poultry dishes.

1½ teaspoons Seasoned Salt (see Index)
1½ teaspoons oregano
½ teaspoon red pepper flakes, optional
1½ teaspoons cumin
1 teaspoon garlic powder
½ teaspoon chili powder
½ teaspoon paprika

Blend all ingredients in small bowl with a fork or spoon.

Store in tightly closed glass jar or spice shaker. Use on grilled chicken or hamburgers.

Makes 2½ Tablespoons

NUTRITIONAL FACTS

*This is considered a **free food** as the carbs are low enough to remain uncalculated.*

TACO SEASONING

2 tablespoons chili powder
2 tablespoons paprika
3 tablespoons cumin
4 tablespoons parsley flakes
2 tablespoons onion powder
1 tablespoon garlic salt
1 tablespoon oregano

Mix all ingredients with fork. Store in tightly covered glass jar or shaker.

Makes 1 Cup

TIPS TO TRY

4 tablespoons mix is equal to the amount in 1 package taco seasoning.

NUTRITIONAL FACTS

*This is considered a **free food** as the carbs are low enough to remain uncalculated.*

ADDITIONAL NUTRITIONAL FACTS

Sausage & Feta Omelet *(pg. 54)*

Serving Size 1 Omelet

Amount per serving:

Calories 396

Total Fat 31.3g

Total Carbohydrate 3g

Dietary Fiber 1g

Sugars 1g

Protein 24.2g

Apple Chips *(pg. 39)*

Serving Size 1/2 Apple

Amount per serving:

Calories 48

Total Fat 0.2g

Total Carbohydrate 12.6g

Dietary Fiber 2g

Sugars 9g

Protein 0.3g

Caramel Apple Dip *(pg. 39)*

Serving Size 1/4 Cup

Amount per serving:

Calories 139

Total Fat 14.6g

Total Carbohydrate 1.9g

Dietary Fiber 0g

Sugars 0g

Protein 0.8g

Southwest Omelet *(pg. 54)*

Serving Size 1 Omelet

Amount per serving:

Calories 232

Total Fat 14.1g

Total Carbohydrate 7.2g

Dietary Fiber 2g

Sugars 1g

Protein 18g

Quesadilla Apple Pie *(pg. 39)*

Serving Size 1/2 Tortilla

Amount per serving:

Calories 128

Total Fat 6.3g

Total Carbohydrate 11.6g

Dietary Fiber 5g

Sugars 4g

Protein 3.1g

Vegetarian Omelet *(pg. 54)*

Serving Size 1 Omelet

Amount per serving:

Calories 215

Total Fat 14.2g

Total Carbohydrate 3.9g

Dietary Fiber 1g

Sugars 2g

Protein 48g

Pizza Burger Panini *(pg. 96)*

Serving Size 1 Panini

Amount per serving:

Calories 487

Total Fat 31.3g

Total Carbohydrate 20.3g

Dietary Fiber 8g

Sugars 4g

Protein 36.6g

Peanut Butter Apple Dip *(pg. 39)*

Serving Size 1/4 Cup

Amount per serving:

Calories 115

Total Fat 8.8g

Total Carbohydrate 4.5g

Dietary Fiber 1g

Sugars 3g

Protein 6.7g

Mediterranean Omelet *(pg. 54)*

Serving Size 1 Omelet

Amount per serving:

Calories 199

Total Fat 13.5g

Total Carbohydrate 2.1g

Dietary Fiber 1g

Sugars 1g

Protein 15.9g

Chicken Bacon Panini *(pg. 96)*

Serving Size 1 Panini

Amount per serving:

Calories 348

Total Fat 19g

Total Carbohydrate 16.3g

Dietary Fiber 7g

Sugars 1g

Protein 32.9g

index

Bake Shop Desserts **133**
Black Bean Brownies 148
Black Bean Fudge Cake 153
Cappuccino Frosting 163
Cappuccino Muffins 139
Chocolate Chip Cookies 136
Chocolate Mocha Cookies 135
Chocolate Mousse 164
Cool Mint Frosting 162
Cream Cheese Frosting 160
Decadent Strawberry Brownie Trifle 146
Dreamsicle Jell-O® Cups 149
Dreamy Fruit Salad 157
Elegant Chocolate Glaze 165
Fudgey Brownies 142
Go Pink! Cupcakes 140
Go Pink! Frosting 161
Mandarin Orange Pudding 151
Power Bars 143
Real Whipped Cream 158
Strawberry Brownie Pizza 145
Sugar Free Mocha Cheesecake 154
Vanilla Pudding 150
Beverages, Hors D'oeuvres & Snacks ... 17
Apple Chips 39
Bacon Wrapped Smokies 20
Caramel Apple Dip 39
Cheese Snack Crackers 29
Cheesy Sausage Balls 28
Cinnamon Tortilla Chips 25
Cinnamon Tortilla Pinwheels 24
Cozy Hot Cocoa 48
Cream Filled Strawberries 36
Eating On The Go 50
For Special Days 50
Frosty Mochaccino 47
Hummus 30
Mini Cheese Balls 27

Peanut Butter Apple Dip 39
Quesadilla Apple Pie 39
Ranch Pecan Snacks 32
Raspberry Lemonade 44
Raspberry Smoothie 42
Raspberry Sweet Tea 43
Snack Ideas 19
Spiced Pecans 35
Strawberry Milkshake 40
Taco Tortilla Pinwheels 23
Toasted Nut Mix 33
Breakfast & Breads **51**
Almond Meal
Dinner Rolls & Bread Crumbs 65
Almond Meal Pancakes 62
Bacon, Egg & Cheese Breakfast Sandwich ... 53
Breakfast Empanadas 58
Coffee Gingerbread Cake 61
Mini Quiche 57
Sunrise Omelets 54
Confectionery **166**
Chocolate Covered Peanut Clusters 168
Chocolate Dipped Strawberries 173
Deluxe Sugar Free Truffles 169
Sugar Free Buckeye Candies 170
Sugar Free Chocolate Chunks 174
Main Dishes & Sides **100**
Baked Chicken Nuggets 102
Burrito Casserole 123
Chicken Fajitas 105
Fajita Marinade For Chicken Or Steak 106
Gourmet Chicken 107
Grilled Asparagus 119
Grilled Dijon Chicken 103
Grilled Fish 128
Grilled Shrimp Scampi 131
Grilled Vegetable Packets 118
Herb Roasted Chicken In Brine 108

Little Cheddar Meat Loaves.........................120
Master Bean Method 114
Mexican Lasagna.....................................122
Oven Broiled Fish....................................132
Quick & Easy Slow Cooker Chicken 110
Refried Beans 115
Savory Lentils...116
Slow Cooker Roast Beef 125
Steaks With Sauce 127
Summertime Barbecued Chicken...............113
Super Chicken & Lentils 111
Sweet & Tangy Barbecued Meatballs 126
Vegetable Stir Fry....................................117

Paninis, Quesadillas & Wraps.............. 89
All-American Hamburgers...........................95
Chicken Quesadillas..................................93
Chicken Salad Tortilla Wraps 97
Cold Cut Wraps 98
Hot Dog Tostados.....................................91
Oven Chicken Quesadillas..........................92
Perfect Paninis...96

Soups & Salads...................................... 66
Angel Fruit Salad......................................74
Cabbage Beef Soup...................................85
Chicken Bacon Chowder 82
Chicken Barley Soup 84
Condensed Mushroom Soup 88
Crispy Tortilla Strips.................................80
Deviled Eggs 79
Finger Jell-O® 75
Quesadilla Salad 70
Rainbow Jell-O® Blocks 76
Ranch Chicken Fajita Salad 68
Souper Duper Chili...................................87
Strawberry Spinach Salad 73
Taco Salad 71
Vegetable Soup 81

The Home Pantry:
Preserves & Mixes 175
Cheese Sauce 177
Fajita Seasoning 185
Herbed Chicken Marinade........................183
Homemade Ketchup 178
Salsa Olé 180

Seasoned Salt...184
Sugar Free Pizza Sauce.............................181
Taco Seasoning.......................................186

SOURCES

BOB'S RED MILL NATURAL FOODS
  13521 SE Pheasant Ct
  Milwaukie, OR 97222
  1-800-349-2173 Toll Free
  www.bobsredmill.com
  xanthan gum

ESSENTIAL EATING SPROUTED FLOURS
  P.O. Box 216
  Mifflinville, PA 18631
  570-586-1557 Phone
  570-586-3112 Fax
  www.essentialeating.com
  certified organic sprouted whole wheat flours

NICKEL MINE HEALTH FOODS
  2123 Mine Rd.
  Paradise, PA 17562
  717-786-1426 Phone
  natural almond meal

SWANSON HEALTH PRODUCTS
  P.O. Box 2803
  Fargo, ND 58108
  1-800-824-4491 Toll Free
  1-800-726-7691 Fax
  www.swansonvitamins.com
  liquid and powdered stevia

NETRITION, INC
  25 Corporate Circle, Suite 118
  Albany, NY 12203
  www.netrition.com
  1-888-817-2411 Toll Free
  518-456-9673 Fax
  EZ Sweetz (liquid sucralose)
  DaVinci® Sugar Free Syrups

ACKNOWLEDGMENTS

First, we thank God, the Giver of life and health to our bodies, for the gift of this diet in controlling seizures in our daughter.

To my husband, James, for being the first one to get the vision for this book, and for encouraging and motivating me in this venture.

To our pediatric neurologist, Dr. Stephen Fulton, MD; for your outstanding expertise, but most of all for your personal attention and interest in Andria's case. None of this would have happened without your advice, support, and excellent hands-on care.

To Rebecca Jennings, MS, RD; for your patience and time in educating us throughout the diet, as well as your personal sacrifice in reviewing all the recipes in this book and calculating the nutritional analysis. Your assistance has been invaluable.

To Beth Zupec-Kania, RD; from the Charlie Foundation, for your time and interest in reviewing this book.

To Michelle Beachy and Christy Smucker, for your awesome photography. Your passion for great food pictures has made this book stunning.

To Karen Miller, for your meticulous editing as you reviewed the text content. Your willingness to take on this project has been a wonderful gift.

To Sharon Miller, Anita Hochstetler, Frieda Mast and Tali Mast for reviewing the rough draft and for your ideas and suggestions.

To Tiffany Reiff, your graphic design work has blown us away. Thank you for sharing our vision and giving our ideas such an amazing look.

To the staff at Carlisle Printing, for helping us navigate the unknown world of publishing.

To our immediate family, for your belief in the success of this work and for your unwavering support and honesty.

To the circle of friends who generously shared, from your personal files, helpful recipes to be adapted for this book.

PHOTOGRAPHY

All the food photographed in this book is authentic and was cooked in my home kitchen. The food has not been artificially glued, sprayed, or colored. Because nothing else has been added, the dishes look the same as they will when you make them.